Raising Your Child Without Milk

Reassuring Advice and Recipes for Parents of Lactose-Intolerant and Milk-Allergic Children

Jane Zukin

PRIMA PUBLISHING

613.26
ZUK

© 1996 by Jane Zukin

PRIMA PUBLISHING and colophon are trademarks of Prima Communications, Inc.

Library of Congress Cataloging-in-Publication Data

Zukin, Jane
  Raising your child without milk : reassuring advice and recipes for parents of lactose-intolerant and milk-allergic children / Jane Zukin
    p.   cm.
  Includes index.
  ISBN 0-7615-0131-2
  1. Lactose intolerance in children—Popular works.   2. Milk-free diet.
3. Milk-free diet—Recipes. I. Title.
RJ399.L33Z85   1995
613.2'6—dc20   95-32000
                                                                         CIP

95 96 97 98 99 AA 10 9 8 7 6 5 4 3 2 1
Printed in the United States of America

How to Order
Single copies may be ordered from Prima Publishing, P.O. Box 1260BK, Rocklin, CA 95677; telephone (916) 632-4400. Quantity discounts are also available. On your letterhead, include information concerning the intended use of the books and the number of books you wish to purchase.

This book is dedicated to my children,
David, Eric, and Renee, who are now all healthy adults
finding their way in the world. My wish for each
of them is a long life of health, happiness, and
security, and I look forward to helping them raise
as many little dairy-sensitive grandchildren
as they choose to give me.

Contents

Introduction

In the little town of Augustov in Lithuania, back before the turn of the century, my grandmother was born and was nursed by her mother and a wet nurse until she was about two years old. Then she was fed a diet that included lots of potatoes, dumplings, stewed vegetables, and braised meats. She was a small woman, my grandmother, only about four foot nine, about the same size as her three brothers and two sisters. But she lived to be about ninety-seven—no one knows her exact age—despite chronic digestive upset, two operations for colon cancer, lifelong high blood pressure, and a stroke in her sixties.

Grama was always a homemaker, but after my grandfather died in 1952 she lived alternately in the homes of her daughters, happily cooking and baking for the family. She was totally dependent upon her children for her support and care. Grama had no stocks or bonds, jewelry or dishes. But she did possess an important family legacy that was passed on to future generations, including my mother, me, and all of my children. That legacy is a dairy sensitivity. And while mother knew that Grama would drink milk in order to relieve her occasional constipation, no one, not even her doctors, ever associated her milk drinking with the chronic digestive upset that plagued her until her death in 1975.

Twenty-five years ago, physical problems associated with milk drinking were not part of medical mainstream thinking. Today things are different. Your family, if it has inherited the legacy of dairy sensitivity as mine has, does not have to helplessly endure illness as a result. Today physicians are better informed and more willing to accept the fact that drinking milk is a problem for a great number of people. The marketplace has responded to recent scientific evidence that millions of Americans and a majority of people across the globe are dairy sensitive by developing a variety of milk-free foods and other products especially for the dairy-sensitive consumer.

My children were raised in a virtually milk-free home, and while they weren't considered exactly "odd" because of it, certainly there were times when others shrugged their shoulders, raised their eyebrows and probably thought we were all just making it up for attention. But your children will be raised in virtually milk-free homes and most people probably will think nothing of it, although there will always be some who will doubt the validity of the food/illness connection.

I have been working my way around milk for over twenty-five years. I have written three books about lactose intolerance and milk allergy before this one, and I publish a national newsletter on the subject. It's curious how something I have been trying to avoid for so long continues to dominate my life. And while right now you may be critically aware of the problems associated with avoiding milk as you try to institute a milk-free lifestyle for your child, eventually, that lifestyle will become easy to live. You will comfortably watch your child grow and thrive despite the elimination of milk from his or her diet. Reassuring you is part of the goal of this book. As I pass on to you the information and practical advice I have garnered as a result of living milk-free for many, many years, my ultimate hope is that any feelings of trepidation or fear you may have for your child's health because he or she is dairy sensitive will be put to rest.

But don't just take my word for it. Dr. Frank O. Oski, director of pediatrics at Johns Hopkins University School of Medicine in Baltimore, states, "Cow's milk is for calves, not for people."

"There are three things you need to know about milk," Oski says. "Number one, nobody needs milk; there are plenty of other sources for everything that milk provides. Number two, certain people are harmed by milk—by allergies, for example. And number three, most people in the world do not drink milk."

Dr. Oski is definitely right. Only in America has the importance of milk been so overemphasized. Dr. Benjamin Spock, perhaps the best known pediatrician in America, has spent a lifetime helping parents make decisions about child rearing. At ninety-one years of age, he has stirred up yet another controversy by urging parents to adopt a diet for their children where meat and milk would be reduced to "something on the order of condiments." Spock is an advocate of a vegetarian diet and argues that the typical American diet consisting of meat and milk is what's killing people. He is convinced that "After the age of three or so, (children) do not need to drink milk and eat dairy products every day."

Dr. Lendon Smith, a nationally respected pediatrician who has written several best-selling books for parents regarding health and nutrition, describes a typical situation that occurs when many nursing mothers wean their infants from breast to bottle:

> Within a month of the switchover to cow's milk (often homogenized and pasteurized) the baby may develop a cold and subsequent bronchial or ear infections, become constipated (cow's milk is the most common cause), or blossom out with an ugly rash of eczema (milk is the prime allergen). It is so clear to me that this sequence represents an allergic response to cow's milk that I have trouble understanding many pediatricians' reluctance to act on this obvious body clue. The cow's milk must be stopped immediately and goat or soy milk substituted, the stress of separation minimized, and sugar in the diet eliminated.

Easy for him to say. You and I both know that sometimes children must be taken off milk. This is not a political statement, but a health fact. However, practically speaking, it isn't always an easy adjustment to make.

Many of my friends and family members are amazed that I continue to write about lactose intolerance and milk allergy after all these years. They often ask me, "What more can you possibly have to say? Don't drink milk. There. That's the book." But, in the case of dairy sensitivity, the obvious solution only provokes more and more questions. In this book, I will try to answer all of your questions. Depending upon the age of your child, some of the information may not apply to your family situation right now, but may give you some insight into the challenges your child will face as he grows or the problems she had earlier that led to her present health condition.

I understand that giving up milk can be difficult for many people because, especially in this country, we have been taught that drinking milk is essential to our health. It is the only food that we have been culturally programmed to revere. And making dramatic lifestyle changes, especially dietary changes that rankle our notions of security and comfort, is not always easy.

When my grandmother came to this country during World War I, she faced immense lifestyle changes. She was afraid to leave home and live in America and never quite got over it. Even after being here for decades, she always longed for the security of the "old country" and especially for the food she ate there, which she always claimed was better than the food in America. Maybe she was right.

1

Why Johnny Can't Drink Milk

Those of you who are reading this book are doing so because your children or grandchildren, or perhaps the children you care for in a school or day-care situation, have been advised that they need to eliminate or restrict milk in their diet. Perhaps you have been given this information after your child was ill or hospitalized, or perhaps you have deduced your child's dairy sensitivity on your own, after seeing how his or her symptoms of milk allergy or intolerance were relieved when you withheld milk and other dairy products. In any case, whether your child is eighteen months old or eighteen years old, rest assured that you are not alone.

I have been in your shoes; as well as being unable to tolerate any dairy foods myself, I have raised three healthy children who are sensitive to milk. Millions of other parents have been in your shoes as well and would like you to know that you *can* raise healthy children in spite of the fact that their dairy intake may have to be limited. We know this because we have lived through it, and so will you and your family. The truth is that millions of children in the world cannot tolerate milk or other dairy foods, so your child is in very good company. I hope that by arming yourself with excellent information and great management ideas, you will feel as confident as I do that your son or daughter will grow up to be just as tall, just as strong, and just as robust as children who do drink milk.

The children in the United States who are growing up without milk and other dairy foods in their diet are doing so not always out of choice, but rather out of necessity. Milk tops the list of the most common allergic offenders for children and is entwined with a variety of other medical conditions that make milk drinking difficult or impossible for children of all ages.

The milk being referred to here is, of course, cow's milk, the stuff American parents think their children should have from day one. But milk is not for everyone, despite what our popular culture may espouse. Milk does not always "do a body good." It is not a *natural*. It is not nature's *perfect food*. In fact, for millions of American children, milk is harmful, unnatural, and highly imperfect. Have we been sold a bill of goods on milk? Possibly. Take a closer look at the facts.

Cow's Milk Is for Calves

Cow's milk comes from female cows. It is the natural food that mother cows provide in order to nurture their calves. In nature, one animal does not suckle another type of animal. Lambs don't nurse from goats, and piglets don't suckle German shepherds. Cow's milk is meant for calves, and it is naturally loaded with the proper nutrients for a bovine baby.

Cow's milk contains approximately 21 percent protein, 45 percent fat, and 34 percent carbohydrate or sugar. Human milk contains 8 percent protein, 55 percent fat, and 37 percent carbohydrate. What's more, the types of proteins and fats found in human and cow's milk are quite different in construction and concentration, making each natural only for its own species. This is a difficult concept for many people in our culture to accept, but it is quite elementary, really. A baby animal is biologically programmed to properly digest the milk of a mother of its own species, not that of another species. Therefore, the assertion that cow's milk is natural for human babies is simply and basically incorrect.

Table 1.1 is a comparison of the nutritive content of human milk, cow's milk, and goat's milk. Take a look at the figures, and notice the similarities and differences. But, as you will see, the figures alone don't tell the whole story.

Table 1.1   Composition of Human, Cow's, and Goat's Milk (per 100 g)*

	HUMAN	COW'S	GOAT'S
Water g	85.2	87.4	87.5
Calories	77	65	67
Protein g	1.1	3.5	3.2
Fat g	4.0	3.5	4.0
Carbohydrate g	9.5	4.9	4.6
Calcium mg	33	118	129
Phosphorus mg	14	93	106
Iron mg	0.1	trace	0.1
Sodium mg	16	50	34
Potassium mg	51	144	180
Vitamin A IU	240	140	160
Thiamine mg	0.01	0.03	0.04
Riboflavin mg	0.04	0.17	0.11
Niacin mg	0.2	0.1	0.3
Vitamin C	5	1	1

*Note: 100 g = almost 1/2 cup
        245 g = 1 cup

Source: U.S. Department of Agriculture

As you can see, human milk has more calories and slightly less water than cow's or goat's milk. The protein content of human milk is about one-third that of cow's or goat's milk and, even more importantly, comprises specifically different proteins. About 60 percent of human milk protein is composed of lactalbumin and the remaining 40 percent is casein. In cow's milk, only 15 percent of the protein is lactalbumin and the remaining 85 percent is casein. While both proteins are normally efficiently digested by babies, human milk with its large concentration of the lactalbumin protein forms fine, fluffy, soft curds, which are digested quite rapidly, while the curd from cow's milk, derived more from the digestion of the protein casein, is larger, tougher, and more slowly digested. Hence, a baby nursed on human milk has loose stools that pass easily and frequently. A baby nursed on cow's milk has harder stools that pass less frequently.

The fats contained in cow's milk, while about the same proportionally as those contained in human milk, comprise a larger amount of short-chain fatty acids, which are somewhat more irritating than the long-chain fatty acids found in human milk. There are additional striking differences between carbohydrate and mineral content of human milk and cow's or goat's milk. Comparatively, human milk contains almost twice as much carbohydrate, or lactose, and profoundly lower amounts of calcium, phosphorus, potassium, and sodium. The lactose in human milk is almost always readily digested by a human baby in the early months, and presumably serves a purpose at its content level. However, the calcium, phosphorus, potassium, and sodium contents found in cow's milk may present—and, in fact, *do* present for many infants—serious health risks because of the baby's inability to properly metabolize such high concentrations of these minerals.

Milk Is Not a Perfect Food

Leaf through many older brochures on health and nutrition and it is quite apparent that, especially during the 1950s, milk became equated with other symbols of "perfect" American life. The photograph of a perfect family dining table showed mom and dad sitting in the dining room or kitchen with a son and a daughter, and a cat and a dog nearby. For breakfast, they ate bacon and eggs, biscuits and butter, orange juice and milk. For dinner, they had meat and potatoes with gravy, salad and peas, bread and butter, and milk. Everyone was smiling, and everyone drank milk. But even if mom and dad chose to drink water or wine instead, it was simply a given that all children had to drink milk with their meals, period. And it was very unusual for a child not to have to finish his or her milk before being served dessert.

Milk was considered basic and essential because it was thought to be the definitive source of protein, vitamins and minerals, and all the other elements required by children to grow. In fact, the book I am looking at right now, which is a nutrition text first published in 1946 and most recently in 1972, contains the following sentences: "There is no adequate substitute for milk. No food has a wider acceptability or offers a greater variety of uses."

Sounds pretty perfect. No "substitute" for it? Those are pretty strong words of praise. But now, fifty years later, we know more about nutrition and that knowledge changes the definition of perfection slightly. Yes, it is true that milk is full of nutrients needed by children who are growing. Milk is an excellent source of calcium, magnesium, and phosphorus for the developing child. It is also an important source of vitamin D for children who do not live in the sunshine states. Vitamin D used to be given to children as cod-liver oil, until someone figured out how to fortify milk with it. Fortified milk became a palatable and easy way to supplement children at risk for developing rickets, a serious, crippling bone disease. In fact, the dramatic reduction, if not elimination, of cases of rickets in America is directly tied to the fortification of whole milk with vitamin D.

But is milk really perfect? Milk lacks two very essential nutrients, iron and vitamin C, both of which are important for developing children. Insufficient amounts of iron in the diet can lead to anemia, and it has long been known that vitamin C is essential for a variety of bodily functions from maintaining healthy gums to fighting infection. Vitamin C is neither made nor stored in the body and must be replaced every single day. To make up for this deficiency, many infants and children take vitamin and mineral supplements in order to receive the full complement of nutrients they require.

Another negative to consider is that milk is a major source of saturated fat in the American diet. One cup of whole milk contains five grams of saturated fat and three grams of unsaturated fat. The same amount of 2-percent milk still contains three grams of saturated fat and two grams of unsaturated fat. We now know that saturated fat contributes to the formation of plaque in the arteries and increases the risk of developing cardiovascular disease, the number one cause of death in America today. Saturated fat in the diet has also been implicated in other health problems, including cancer of the colon and breast.

Because some scientific studies have shown that children fed skim milk or 1-percent milk may not be receiving an adequate caloric intake and are at risk for poor physical development, most health-care givers advise that very young children drink either whole or 2-percent milk. If this recommendation is followed, consider the saturated fat intake of those children who diligently drink three or four cups of milk per day: They will be taking in about twelve to twenty grams of saturated fat, which is about equivalent to eating three to four tablespoons of lard each and every day. In light of what we know today about saturated fat in the diet, you tell me how this practice can be justified.

As for protein, one cup of milk contains nine grams of protein, about the same amount as a hamburger. Yet recently government panels have discovered that Americans eat far too much protein on a regular basis, and the latest recommendations call for only eighteen to twenty grams of protein per day for children four years old and under. What this means, then, is that the child who is drinking three or four cups of milk per day is being given twenty-seven to thirty-six grams of protein from the milk alone. If the child also eats one egg at six grams of protein, two tablespoons of peanut butter at eight grams of protein, and two chicken drumsticks at twenty-four grams of protein, that child will now be eating sixty-five to seventy-four grams of protein per day, over three times the recommended daily allowance!

So, while many dairy associations tout their products as "perfect," clearly, perfection, if it means a quintessentially good food source of vitamins, minerals, proteins, and fats, is not the proper definition of milk. Proof of this is the recent demotion of milk in the newly designed food pyramid. For many years, we were taught about the four food groups. The milk group was always depicted at the top of the diagram, indicating its preeminence and importance. Recent research, however, has led to the development of the food pyramid (discussed more fully in Chapter 2), which finds the milk group lowered in status considerably.

Milk Is Not for Everyone

We've all heard the ads: "Milk is for everyone." "Milk does a body good." The dairy industry is a major economic force in the United States, with countless associations, councils, boards, and lobbyists, all working toward one end—the promotion of dairy products. The dairy industry is a "super-marketer" of milk and other dairy foods to the American people. While most people are probably unaware of the Prune Board or the Yogurt Association, or perhaps even the Pork Producers of America, almost everyone has heard of the Dairy Council, or if not, at least everyone is familiar with the message of the Dairy Council and its associated organizations. The benefits of drinking milk are reiterated for the American people in print, on billboards, on the radio, on television, even in movie theaters. As a culture, we are inundated with messages about the importance of drinking milk. And, as a culture, we believe every word.

But there are many people in this country and, indeed, around the world for whom drinking milk is not a good idea. In fact, studies have shown that over half of the world's population is unable to drink milk due to an intolerance of the carbohydrate in milk—lactose. Furthermore, people with other medical conditions such as celiac disease, cancer, and even those struck down by the flu, to name just a few, are often medically unable to tolerate milk. While doctors know that this is the case, it is generally very difficult for physicians to advise their patients to cut back on their milk consumption, or for patients to actually accept this treatment, because drinking milk and the positive associations that accompany the practice are so heavily ingrained in our attitudes. Some physicians are actually afraid to advise against drinking milk, even though they know that some of their patients have health problems associated with it.

Tantamount to a sort of "milk worship," the level of importance given to milk drinking in western society is a recent phenomenon, historically speaking. Only in the past ten thousand years has milk been utilized as a food beyond infancy. In most societies, infants were fed on breast milk until about the age of two or three. After that, there was no drinking of milk. It is only in the modern western world that the practice of milk drinking extends beyond that time, into adulthood.

Geographers and anthropologists explain that during the hunting and gathering stage of evolution, there were no domesticated animals to be milked. The evidence indicates that it was not until between 4000 and 3000 B.C. that animals were milked in northern Africa and southwest Asia, although dairying was not a widespread practice. Moving forward to A.D. 1500, evidence of nondairying cultures is still more prevalent than that of dairying cultures, even throughout the regions of European expansion and development. Studies have shown that the bulk of African people, Asian people (including the people of Korea, China, and Vietnam), Pacific Islanders, and people from North and South America did not drink milk after weaning, perhaps because dairying was slow to develop. It was, in many cases, impractical and unsuited to the environment.

European explorers, during the great era of discovery, observed that most of the nondairying cultures they encountered considered the manipulation of animal udders to be unnatural and forbidden. Religious practices came into play as well. Asian cultures believed in the concept of "ahimsa," or nonviolence to every living being. Because these people believed that taking animal milk for a human was robbing the animal young of its rightful nourishment, they did not milk animals.

Quite curiously, there is also recorded evidence of people who were opposed to drinking milk because they felt that it caused them symptoms of stomach cramps, gas, nausea, and vomiting. At the time, European travelers who recorded their encounters with other cultures considered these symptoms to be psychosomatic, caused by an aversion to drinking milk. Even though we now know that these symptoms are completely physical, based on the malabsorption of lactose, attitudes passed on from generation to generation are often very difficult to change.

In 1979, a lawsuit was brought by the Federal Trade Commission (FTC) against the State of California Milk Producers Advisory Board. The FTC complained that the use of an advertising slogan "Everybody needs milk" was "unfair, false, misleading and deceptive." The FTC case was based on the contention that large numbers of people did not need milk because they were either lactose intolerant or had a milk allergy.

The judge, Daniel H. Hanscomb, after hearing thirty-five expert witnesses, decided that there was an insignificant clinical threat to the health of individuals due to milk drinking. In the ruling, Judge Hanscomb asserted that "The weight of the scientific and medical evidence established that milk in moderate amounts at a time was not detrimental but beneficial, even for people who could not digest lactose in milk. They benefited from all the other nutrients essential for a good diet."

He went on to state that "Milk is one of the most nutritious foods in the nation's diet, and from the standpoint of the population as a whole, or even significant population groups, is literally 'essential, necessary and needed.' The withdrawal of milk from any major population group would amount to a nutritional disaster."

A "nutritional disaster"? It would be very interesting to see what would happen if the same lawsuit were brought today. It is hard to believe that the American consumer, more sophisticated about nutrition than ever before, would stand for the warped legal logic of the claim that eating food that makes you sick is good for you. Believe me, no food is that sacred. *Not even milk.*

Today, we know that there are many valid medical reasons for children to abstain from drinking milk and there is a wide variety of other food choices and supplement options available to give children the nutrition they need to grow up healthfully.

With education and support, parents and caretakers of children who must restrict or eliminate milk and other dairy foods can learn how to raise healthy children without milk. And as you join the rest of us who are coping every day with a dairy-free lifestyle, you will learn to feel confident in your ability to do so.

Lactose Intolerance

One of the major components of all animal milk is its carbohydrate or sugar, called *lactose*. Lactose is a disaccharide—a double sugar—composed of glucose and galactose. During the first phase of digestion, lactose must be split into its two component sugars. The glucose component is then sent into the bloodstream and the galactose is sent to the liver where it is hydrolyzed (converted) into glucose.

In order to begin the process of digesting lactose, the body requires a specific enzyme called *lactase* to perform the initial phase of hydrolysis. The lactase enzyme is located in the small intestine, specifically attached to the brush border or villi at the surface of the intestinal epithelial cells. It is one of many enzymes that are responsible for the digestion of sugars and is generally present in large quantities at birth.

Lactose digestion is directly dependent upon the ratio of lactose ingested to lactase enzyme present. If there is an insufficient amount of lactase enzyme, unabsorbed lactose remains in the small intestine where it causes an osmotic effect, that is, it draws water into the area and retains it. Unabsorbed lactose may also increase the motility of the gastrointestional tract, causing the intestinal contents to move more rapidly than usual. When the unmetabolized lactose passes farther down into the colon, it becomes a target of bacterial fermentation. The normal bacteria present in the colon break down the lactose into hydrogen, carbon dioxide, and lactic acid. The osmotic, or water, pressure increases again, and the cells of the colon secrete more fluid. The result of the bacterial fermentation is gas, pain, and diarrhea.

Studies of lactose intolerance have revealed without a doubt that while nearly all infants are born with high lactase enzyme levels, there is a marked drop in enzyme production between the ages of two and three among most children in the world. This reduction generally continues through the teenage years and into adulthood, accounting for the fact that most adults in the world have very low lactase enzyme levels compared to their levels at birth. It is normal and natural for people to experience lowering lactase enzyme levels throughout their lives. In fact, researchers hypothesize that people who can comfortably digest milk through adulthood are actually able to do so as a result of a mutated gene. Lactose intolerance, therefore, is the norm, while lactose tolerance is the mutation.

The study of lactose intolerance has yielded some very important results, including the categorizing of the condition into three different medical scenarios. They are *primary lactose intolerance, secondary lactose intolerance,* and *alactasia.*

Primary Lactose Intolerance

Primary lactose intolerance is an inherited, age-related reduction in lactase enzyme activity. Studies of families from a variety of ethnic groups have shown that lactose absorption is inherited as an autosomal dominant characteristic. In other words, if your child is lactose intolerant, he or she has probably inherited the condition from you or someone else in your family. Lactose intolerance is highly subjective, highly individualized. Different people have different lactase enzyme levels, different degrees of enzyme efficiency, and different thresholds of tolerance. In addition, other factors, such as the amount of milk ingested, the type of dairy food eaten, the manner in which the lactose is consumed (drinking milk alone or with other foods), the ability of the colon to handle excess fluids, the time taken for gastric emptying, and the action of certain hormones, affect the symptomatic response to undigested lactose in various people with lactose intolerance.

According to a number of studies examined in the *American Journal of Clinical Nutrition* in 1988, the incidence of primary lactose intolerance is high in the majority of people, with the exception of those of northern European descent. In North America, lactose intolerance is found in about 79 percent of American Indians, 75 percent of African Americans, 51 percent of Hispanics, and 21 percent of Caucasians. Other studies conducted by Dr. Theodore Bayless of Johns Hopkins University and his colleagues have found that the great majority of Asians, Africans, Italians, Greeks, and Jews of both eastern European and Mediterranean descent retain very little lactase enzyme as adults, perhaps losing as much as 90 to 99 percent of their enzyme activity with age.

Lactose intolerance was first formally identified in 1907 as the result of work done by biochemist Lafayette B. Mendel. However, the study of lactose intolerance did not become popular again until nearly sixty years later. From the late 1960s into the late 1970s a variety of studies were done indicating the high prevalence of lactose malabsorption in children throughout the world.

One significant study, which was conducted by David M. Paige, M.D., in 1977, involved over four hundred African American children in Baltimore and determined the percentages of lactose malabsorbers across an age span from thirteen months to twelve years of age. The results confirmed lactose intolerance in approximately 27 percent of the one- to two-year-olds; 33 percent of the five- to six-year-olds; and 74 percent of the eleven- to twelve-year-olds. There was no difference between boys and girls nor across socioeconomic groups. A parallel study of Caucasian children showed that 17 perent were malabsorbers between the ages of one to twelve years.

Further studies conducted by Dr. Bayless attempted to identify percentages of lactose intolerance found in a variety of ethnic groups around the globe. The results of this study, depicted in Table 1.2, indicate the genetic background that accounts for the presence of the lactose intolerance. Where is your family in this ethnically diverse look at the prevalence of inherited primary lactose intolerance? Is your heritage Greek or Japanese or Colombian? Are you African American or Jewish? Your family tree

Table 1.2 Prevalence of Lactose Intolerance Among Adults

African Americans	70%
American Indians	85%
Arabs	80%
Ashkenazi Jews	78%
Colombian Indians	57%
Danish	4%
Filipinos	93%
Finns	18%
Greek Cypriots	87%
Greenland Eskimos	87%
Indians	55%
Israeli Jews	63%
Japanese	92%
Mexican Americans	60%
Peruvians	64%
Swiss	8%
Thai	94%
White Americans	9%

Source: Theodore M. Bayless, M.D., Johns Hopkins University Hospital Practice, October 1976

helps determine the probability of your child being lactose intolerant, perhaps as an infant, perhaps not until six years of age, perhaps not until eighteen. But if the ethnic heritage is there, the results of the genetic factors at work will eventually follow.

From the information gathered in this study, Dr. Bayless was able to extrapolate numbers regarding lactose intolerance in the United States. He estimated that at least 30 million people in the United States were lactose intolerant at the time. This figure includes an estimated 16 million adults and teenagers of Northern European descent, 2.4 million Jewish adults and teenagers, and 800,000 elementary-school-aged children. Today, the numbers are significantly higher since the population of the United States has grown markedly in the almost twenty years that have passed since Dr. Bayless drew these conclusions. Similar large population studies of people in the United States, which could yield more exact figures, have not been done since then.

Secondary Lactose Intolerance

Secondary lactose intolerance is an acquired lactose intolerance not necessarily programmed by genetics. Because the lactase enzyme is directly responsible for the digestion of lactose, any condition that diminishes or impairs the ability of the enzyme to do its job will result in undigested lactose in the gut. Now, think of the myriad medical conditions that affect the small intestine: They vary from a passing virus to influenza to Crohn's disease to cancer. A one-day bout with diarrhea itself can deplete the small intestine of lactase enzyme.

The main difference between primary and secondary lactose intolerance, however, is the fact that people in the throes of an episode of secondary lactose intolerance will soon regain their ability to digest lactose when the assaulted intestinal area heals, or otherwise returns to normal, although it is possible to acquire permanent lactose intolerance as a secondary condition from surgery or chronic disease. An example of the latter is a seventeen-year-old girl with Crohn's disease who requires surgery to remove all or part of the small intestine. When her disease was active, she may have had only occasional bouts with secondary lactose intolerance during a flare-up of the Crohn's disease, but after surgery, she may be permanently lactose intolerant due to the total absence of enzyme located in the small intestine, which was permanently removed.

A more typical example of secondary lactose intolerance is the child who becomes sick with a cold or flu and has diarrhea for a few days. Because of the diarrhea, that child is unable to digest dairy foods during the run of the cold, but will be back to his or her normal level of lactose digestion within a few days. For this reason, many pediatricians now recommend that teething infants, who are so often susceptible to digestive distress, refrain from cow's milk formula during the teething episode and instead be temporarily switched to a soy formula.

It is easy to understand why refraining from dairy foods during a limited period of secondary lactose intolerance is necessary and wise: Continuing to offend a lactase enzyme–reduced gut will only prolong the discomfort and make matters worse.

See the box following for a partial list of medical conditions that may cause or contribute to secondary lactose intolerance in infants and children. Some of them will be discussed in greater detail later in this chapter.

Drugs may be another cause of secondary lactose intolerance. Specifically, laxatives, antacids with magnesia, and antibiotics are among some of the offenders for infants and children. Children undergoing chemotherapy are also at risk for developing secondary lactose intolerance. The same is true for children undergoing abdominal radiation. Besides injury to the intestine, a side effect of these therapies is often diarrhea, which depletes the lactase enzyme and makes children undergoing these treatments temporarily lactose intolerant. Eliminating milk and other dairy foods from their diet during treatment is usually standard practice. These children are usually given predigested hypoallergenic formulas or enzyme-treated milks instead.

Alactasia

Alactasia is a rare congenital abnormality seen in infants. In this case, the infant is born without sufficient lactase enzyme to digest either breast or cow's milk. Alactasia can be fatal if not recognized promptly. The symptoms of alactasia include abdominal pain, abdominal distension, and watery diarrhea. The pH of the stools is usually low, indicating high acidity, due to the bacterial fermentation in the baby's gut. Without prompt treatment, malnutrition will ensue.

Some Causes of Secondary Lactose Intolerance

Viruses

Influenza

Crohn's disease

Ulcerative colitis

Celiac disease

Gastroenteritis

Kwashiorkor (a type of malnutrition)

Hyperthyroidism

Irritable bowel syndrome

Galactosemia (a congenital abnormality)

Prematurity

Bacterial infections including those from *Salmonella, E. Coli, Shigella, Giardia,* or other parasites

Infectious hepatitis

Milk-protein allergy

Recurrent abdominal pain syndrome

Personally, I had three babies born with unusually low lactase enzyme levels. Each one exhibited symptoms of severe lactose intolerance within the first seven to ten days of life. When my first child, David, was born in 1971, it took almost three months to make the diagnosis. By the time Eric was born in 1972, he was diagnosed at two weeks. In 1976 when my daughter, Renee, was born, she was immediately placed on soy formula in the hospital nursery.

Today, there is more information available to health-care providers about cow's milk intolerance and breast-feeding problems than there was twenty-five years ago. And there are certainly much better feeding options for these infants today. In 1971, alternative soy formulas were about the only practical choice, and they had to be special-ordered from the pharmacy. Some critically ill infants with milk intolerance were fed on banana milk, meat-based formulas, or almond milks. I actually knew of a family whose infant daughter was being nursed on 7Up for a considerable time. Luckily for infants with alactasia today, prehydrolyzed formulas are as easy to come by as a glass of chocolate milk.

Furthermore, pediatricians are much more likely to switch an infant's formula today than was the case years ago. The prevailing theory at that time was that some discomfort might be better than tampering with a baby's "lifeblood." After all, twenty-five years ago, pediatricians thought that infants had limited feelings of pain and that wailing was simply a part of their maturing nervous system.

When I think back to David's first months, I wonder how we let the weeks slip by without doing something more constructive. My infant son screamed so, barely slept, and had projectile vomiting and explosive diarrhea. He usually gulped and gasped when he drank his formula and fought with the nipple being offered to him. He was eventually sedated, and after many diagnostic tests and much effort to comfort him, he was finally switched to a soy formula. His first feeding was miraculous in that he actually lay back, relaxed, and nursed peacefully. I believe that my baby had been trying to tell us something very important all along, but we were not paying close enough attention thanks to our own inexperience as parents and, in part, to a medical community that was ill-informed. Luckily, health care for infants with alactasia is much better today.

Alactasia may not always be the culprit in very sick, lactose-intolerant infants. Some infants who present with lactose intolerance may do so as the result of having had gastroenteritis, which has damaged the intestinal mucosa. The gastroenteritis may be the result of either a viral or bacterial infection or some other medical problem. Today, precise diagnosis of alactasia is made through a biopsy technique, but because of its invasive nature, this procedure is not usually done on infants unless necessary for clinical testing to determine other digestive diseases or to detect obstructions. Biopsy clearly may not be required if a switch in the infant's formula fixes the problem.

While it may not always be clear whether the lactose-intolerant infant is suffering from alactasia, early primary lactose intolerance, or secondary lactose intolerance due to gastroenteritis, at least parents can take comfort in knowing that there are viable and healthy feeding options available to babies who cannot tolerate breast or cow's milk, and today there are knowledgeable pediatricians willing to prescribe them.

Preterm Infants

As mentioned before, all the various carbohydrates require specific enzymes for hydrolysis. Sucrose requires the sucrase enzyme, maltose requires the maltase enzyme, and lactose requires the lactase enzyme. Premature infants, depending upon their age at birth, may not possess the full complement of digestive enzymes, making hydrolysis of carbohydrates difficult or impossible.

It is known that some enzymes, sucrase and maltase specifically, do reach their peak prenatally. However, the lactase enzyme develops late in the gestation period, really just before the baby's birth, making it very tricky for a premature infant to have enough enzyme necessary to digest milk well. Also, the lactase enzyme is much more easily damaged than the others. Therefore, premature infants are usually routinely placed on prehydrolyzed formulas in which the carbohydrates and proteins have been metabolized before ingestion. Premature infants, depending upon their age at birth and, of course, their physical condition, will require very specific feeding instructions from a pediatrician. Altering your premature infant's diet on your own is not recommended.

Testing for Lactose Intolerance

There are several diagnostic tests that can be administered to help verify the existence of lactose intolerance. Your child's pediatrician will make the determination as to which test is appropriate for your child.

Home Testing   The simplest test for lactose intolerance can be done at home, although it can only practically be used for children about two years old or older. While not clinically accurate, home testing can give you some idea of your child's level of lactose intolerance. The procedure involves first eliminating all sources of lactose and then reintroducing milk as a challenge. To do this, start by eliminating all dairy products and other food items containing lactose for one week. Then give your child a tall glass of milk. If digestive distress symptoms of lactose intolerance occur within three hours of drinking the milk, you know for certain that your child has some degree of lactose intolerance. Usually, the cramping and diarrhea will start within the first hour of drinking the milk, but not always. Determining your child's specific lactose-tolerance level and appropriate feeding regimen will be discussed more completely in Chapter 4. In the case of infants, an easy way to discover lactose intolerance is to simply substitute a lactose-free formula for milk and watch to see if the baby's symptoms of gas and diarrhea abate. Check with your child's pediatrician for further advice.

There are several medical tests used to clinically determine lactose intolerance that your child's pediatrician may want to order. The precise test chosen will depend upon your child's age and general physical condition. Infants may be given a stool acidity test and older children will most likely be given either a lactose tolerance test or a hydrogen breath test.

Lactose Tolerance Test   When lactose is properly broken down in the digestive tract by the lactase enzyme, it is split into its two component sugars—glucose and galactose. From there, the liver breaks down the galactose further, to yield glucose as well. The glucose produced by digestion enters the bloodstream and can be measured there. Should there be no rise in blood glucose levels or only a nominal rise in blood glucose levels after ingesting lactose, complete hydrolysis did not occur.

Practically, what this means is that during the lactose tolerance test, the child will fast for a designated period of time. He or she will have blood drawn to measure the fasting glucose level. Then, the child will be given a precise amount of lemonade or other such drink containing a measured amount of lactose, based on the child's weight. Over the next two hours, usually during thirty-minute intervals, the child will have his or her blood drawn, and glucose levels will be measured. If the glucose level rises in the blood sufficiently, it is evidence of absorption. If the glucose level fails to rise, it is conclusive proof of lactose intolerance.

Lactose-intolerant children being given this test are highly likely to experience some pain, cramping, and diarrhea during the test because of drinking the lactose load. In fact, these symptoms are specifically noted during the test and are further evidence of the lactose-intolerant diagnosis. For the comfort of the child, the lactose load should be adjusted in relation to the child's weight, but parents and children should be aware that there will most likely be some discomfort during the test and afterward.

Hydrogen Breath Test   Another test commonly given to children to determine lactose intolerance is the hydrogen breath test. This test measures the amount of hydrogen expressed through the lungs as a result of undigested lactose in the gut. The advantage to this test for many is the fact that no needles are involved. For that reason, it is usually preferred by pediatricians as a means of diagnosing children.

Normally, we have very little, almost no, hydrogen in our breath. But, when lactose is not properly hydrolyzed in the small intestine, it moves into the colon and is fermented by the bacteria there. This fermentation yields several gasses, one of which is hydrogen. The hydrogen is then expelled through our lungs in our breath and can be measured as a diagnostic tool.

Practically, this test is very similar to the lactose tolerance test in its procedure. After a fasting period, the child has his or her breath measured for hydrogen. Then, after drinking a lactose load, the hydrogen in the breath is measured again, usually over the course of two hours. Should the hydrogen level in the breath rise, it reveals undigested lactose in the colon and a lactose-intolerance diagnosis is confirmed. Again, the child will experience digestive distress during and after the test.

Stool Acidity Test   This test for lactose intolerance is generally used to make the diagnosis in infants and toddlers because it is completely noninvasive and requires absolutely no cooperation from the child. When undigested lactose reaches the colon, the bacteria present ferment it. Aside from hydrogen, lactic acid and other short-chain fatty acids will be produced.

Excesses of these acids will be present in the stool and can be measured. If the acidity of the stool is higher than normal, lactose intolerance is positively identified. Usually, there is excess glucose in the stool as well. It too, can be measured. Infants who are breast-fed will have elevated acid levels in their stool, but this can be accounted for in the test situation.

Urine Test   It is possible for undigested lactose to show up in the urine and be measured there. However, this test can yield false positives for other reasons, and it is usually not relied upon for accurate lactose-intolerance diagnosis. Lactosuria, a spilling of lactose into the urine can also be caused by hyperthyroidism, Crohn's disease, nontropical sprue, or breast-feeding.

Galactose Test   This test measures galactose in the bloodstream. When lactose is split into its two component sugars, glucose and galactose, the galactose travels through the bloodstream to the liver for conversion into glucose. It has been found that ethanol delays conversion of galactose to glucose and a measurement can be determined. But because the test relies on the use of alcohol and blood extraction, it is not recommended for children.

Biopsy   Direct measurement of the lactase enzyme level in the small intestine is possible through intestinal intubation and biopsy. This is actually the most precise measurement of all. However, for a variety of reasons including the highly disadvantageous use of an invasive procedure, unless done as part of another diagnostic test, it is not used to determine lactose intolerance in infants or children.

Milk-Protein Allergy

Not to be confused with lactose intolerance, a *milk-protein allergy* is a completely different medical condition that requires different feeding treatment for infants and children (see Table 1.3). A milk-protein allergy is an immunological response to protein that passes through the intestinal walls and into the bloodstream unaffected by hydrolysis. In other words, the protein enters the bloodstream whole, undigested. In the blood of an allergic infant, child, or adult, the milk protein is perceived as an *allergen,* an offensive molecule that incites the body's immune response to kick into gear and purge itself of the offender by producing antibodies in the bloodstream and other physical responses. Milk-protein allergy usually presents in infants three to six months old and younger, although it has been known to present at any time throughout a person's life.

Milk-protein-allergic infants and children have a myriad of symptoms depending upon their individual immune system. Some immune responses that may occur include vomiting, diarrhea, urticaria (hives), rash, cough, rhinitis (runny nose), swelling of the skin, asthma, and even death. You could probably recognize some of the most familiar allergic reactions to milk protein in infants and children you know. Some of the signs have become so well-known, they have names such as:

- The allergic shiner—dark circles around the eyes of youngsters caused by pooling blood in the eye area
- The allergic salute—a crinkled top of the nose caused by the child constantly pushing upward on an itchy nose

Table 1.3   Lactose Intolerance and Milk Allergy
Similarities and Differences

	LACTOSE INTOLERANCE	MILK ALLERGY
Age of onset	Usually after age 2	Early infancy
Dairy factor	Milk sugar	Milk protein
Cause	Inherited/Acquired	Inherited/Acquired
Symptoms include:		
Diarrhea	Yes	Yes
Vomiting	Yes	Yes
Abdominal pain	Yes	Yes
Abdominal bloating	Yes	Yes
Skin rash	No	Yes
Runny nose	No	Yes
Asthma	No	Yes
Hives	No	Yes
Anaphylaxis	No	Yes
Duration	Indefinite	Late childhood
Treatment	Restriction of lactose including whey	Restriction of whey, casein, lactalbumin, and lactoglobulin

- Hot cheeks—bright red cheeks caused by inflammation
- Bright red ears—ears are notorious for inflammation in allergic children

Milk-protein allergy has been implicated in a variety of negative responses in children from hyperactivity to bed-wetting to ticklishness. These signs of hypersensitivity may indicate an immune system on alert.

In a paper referenced in the *American Journal of Clinical Nutrition* published in 1988, data reported on symptoms of milk-protein allergy produced these results: In 88 percent of cases, diarrhea was reported; in 44 percent of cases, vomiting was reported; in 39 percent of cases, abdominal pain was reported; in 33 percent of cases, atopic dermatitis was reported; in 31 percent of cases, rhinitis was reported; in 31 percent of cases, asthma was reported; in 13 percent of cases, urticaria was reported; and in 12 percent of cases, anaphylaxis (a life-threatening reaction) was reported.

Several of my readers have told me that their children are so sensitive to milk that even if they touch milk, it will cause a reaction. One mother in California related how her husband ate a bowl of oatmeal topped with milk every single morning. Each time he quickly kissed their baby good-bye, a red welt in the shape of his kiss would appear on the baby's cheek!

The exact number of older children and adults who are allergic to cow's milk is not well determined. Some sources doubt the existence of cow's milk allergy in teenagers and adults, while other experts maintain the condition may persist throughout life. But it has been documented that some adults sensitive to cow's milk protein may also have an allergic reaction to all beef products and often eggs as well. Children with cow's milk–protein allergy are often allergic to other foods, which could include eggs, wheat, or corn.

While the numbers are difficult to confirm, recent research indicates that cow's milk–protein allergy is probably not as prevalent as was once thought, but rather affects perhaps 3 to 7 percent of infants. It is, however, the number one allergy in infants because cow's milk is the basis of almost all commercial formulas given to infants today; it is basically their complete diet for months.

Even breast milk may pose a problem for some infants highly reactive to cow's milk protein. While there has never been clinical evidence of any allergic reaction to breast milk protein in infants, it has been shown that nursing mothers who drink milk pass those cow's milk proteins through their breast milk on to their infants, who may then have an allergic reaction. As mothers are apt to consume more milk and other dairy foods for added calcium during the nursing period, this may pose a problem for some babies. The mother's restriction or elimination of milk in her diet, however, has been proven definitively to have a beneficial effect on those breast-fed infants with a milk-protein allergy. If breast-feeding mothers are unaware of this fact, they may be unknowingly precipitating allergic symptoms in their infants, which could be eliminated by a simple decrease in their own dairy intake.

Recently, there has been a controversy brewing over the role of cow's milk–protein allergy and the development of juvenile diabetes. A study reported in the *Annals of Medicine,* October 1991, was conducted by researchers at the Hospital for Sick Children in Toronto, Ontario. The study drew the conclusion that the protein bovine serum albumin might be an important environmental factor in the immune response that causes insulin-dependent diabetes in children genetically predisposed to the disease. While this one study does not present a hard-and-fast conclusion, parents of children with juvenile diabetes or families with a history of juvenile diabetes will want to get appropriate advice from medical specialists before feeding their infants and young children a diet laden with cow's milk.

There are approximately twenty different proteins in cow's milk, and a very complex system is in place in the body for the efficient and complete digestion of those proteins. But sometimes, problems do occur. The proteins that seem to cause the most difficulty include *casein,* which is found in the curd of the milk when separated as in cheese making, and the whey proteins, *lactalbumin* and *lactoglobulin,* which travel with lactose to the watery portion of the milk during separation. All of these proteins are contained in fluid cow's milk and cow's milk formula.

A serious negative effect of undigested cow's milk protein in the gut is the damage it does to the intestinal mucosa. Biopsies have revealed that the intestinal linings of patients with milk-protein allergy are riddled with lesions and partial atrophy of the intestinal villi. Remembering that it is precisely these intestinal villi that hold the digestive enzymes, specifically lactase, it is easy then to understand how a milk-protein allergy can cause a secondary lactose intolerance by damaging the intestinal areas that house the lactase enzyme. If left untreated, infants and children with milk-protein allergy will become lactose intolerant over time, perhaps permanently.

The course of severity for a milk-protein allergy is the reverse of lactose intolerance. As we have seen, the body's lactase enzyme production wanes with time, causing more intolerance as people grow and age. The exact opposite is true of milk-protein allergy. Because milk allergy evokes an immune response, as the infant or young child grows he or she will experience a maturation of the digestive system and the immune system resulting in fewer milk-protein allergens penetrating the mucosa of the intestine. This happens most often between the ages of one and four. But until the allergy has been outgrown, strict avoidance of cow's milk is the recommended treatment. Approximately 25 percent of infants and young children with cow's milk–protein allergy are also sensitive to soy protein, so special attention must be paid to the child's alternative formula or milk substitute as well.

Testing for Milk-Protein Allergy

Clinical testing for milk-protein allergy is not well established. The most reliable testing method is the challenge test in which a quantity of milk is given, the resulting allergic symptoms noted, the milk is removed from the diet while symptoms abate, and then reintroduced as a challenge in order to positively verify the allergy when symptoms recur. However, *and this is imperative,* because the condition usually appears in babies and because babies have been known to experience catastrophic and even life-threatening effects from early reintroduction of cow's milk as a challenge, infants are generally never challenged before twenty-four months, and only under a doctor's supervision. If challenged too early, some infants and young children become irreversibly allergic and run the risk of serious medical complications. Therefore, when milk-protein allergy is diagnosed in infants, the standard treatment is generally soy or another alternative formula along with strict avoidance of milk and other dairy foods until at least two years of age. Many pediatricians recommend avoidance until four or five years of age.

Other testing methods for milk-protein allergy offer very mixed and not terribly reliable results. One test often given to young children is the radioallergosorbent test or RAST. This blood test has been reviewed by many researchers for its reliability with respect to milk protein, but in a complete study of diagnostic methods for determining milk-protein allergy reported in *Milk Intolerances and Rejection,* 1983, Karger and Basel, the scientists conclude that:

> Serum anti-milk IgE antibodies are usually detected by RAST, unfortunately their presence is neither specific nor constant. One of the reasons for the poor diagnostic abilities of RAST is probably due to the large number of antigens, at least 30 for cow's milk, in the dietary extracts used. In addition, anti-milk IgE may be found without milk allergy in celiac disease and in blind loops, gastrointestinal fistulas, and false passages containing milk. . . . On the contrary, RAST . . . were found to be highly reliable for the diagnosis of allergy to cod fish, peas, nuts, peanuts, and egg white.

Skin tests yield about the same mediocre reliability for cow's milk–protein allergy as RAST. Another type of diagnostic test is the immune complex hypersensitivity (type III), which was reviewed in the same study with the following results:

> The finding of precipitating anti-milk antibodies has no diagnostic value, since these antibodies are very common in the normal infant and they are found in similar tiers in milk allergy and other diseases such as celiac disease, IgE deficiency and the recovery phase of acute gastroenteritis.

Therefore, the general medical consensus is that standard diagnostic allergy tests are not recommended for milk allergy, and especially not in children. Parents need not demand such tests be done for milk allergy nor think a physician better qualified for ordering them. On the contrary, most pediatric allergists do not rely on such tests for positive identification of cow's milk–protein allergy.

A simple test for milk-protein allergy recommended by Johns Hopkins gastroenterologist Dr. Theodore Bayless is done through the elimination of lactose intolerance as a diagnosis using the stool acidity test discussed above. Considering that milk is the main food of the infant, a child with vomiting or diarrhea or eczema, who does not have other congenital or malabsorption diseases as determined through medical testing, could be definitively diagnosed with milk allergy by ruling out lactose intolerance through a test measuring acid in the stool, as discussed in the section on lactose intolerance. The logic is easy to follow. The infant who presents with symptoms that could be either lactose intolerance or milk allergy can be positively diagnosed as being allergic to milk if he or she is not lactose intolerant.

There are a number of allergy testing methods being practiced at various clinics around the country that do not have the sanction of the American Board of Allergy and Immunology for validity or effectiveness. These tests are not considered legitimate diagnostic tools by the medical profession because they have not been scientifically or rigorously tested. These tests require cytotoxic testing, which involves adding extracts of specific foods to a sample of the patient's blood; provocation and neutralization testing, which involves administering extracts of foods under the skin or tongue; skin titration (Rinkel method), which involves injecting suspected allergens; urine autoinjection, which involves injecting sterilized urine into muscle; and clinical ecology and allergy analysis by mail.

Celiac Disease

Strictly speaking, there are several diseases that involve a "celiac syndrome," that is, the malabsorption of gluten accompanied by nutritional deficiencies. They are gluten-induced enteropathy, also known as primary idiopathic steatorrhea; celiac disease (in children); nontropical sprue (in adults); cystic fibrosis; and kwash-iorkor. In all of these diseases, adults or children cannot digest gluten, the protein in wheat and some other grains as well. Children with celiac disease will see the onset of symptoms develop slowly, insidiously. The "celiac" child will have diarrhea, steatorrhea (excessive amount of fat in the stool), weight loss, and a pale, frothy stool. He or she may be irritable and have frequent bouts of vomiting. Infants with celiac disease may present with failure to thrive. There may be blood in the stool as well as reduced calcium levels in the bloodstream. In a recent study reported in *Nutrition in Pediatrics* by W. Allan Walker, M.D., and John B. Watkins, M.D., more than 30 percent of babies under twelve months old with intractable diarrhea were found to have celiac disease.

The intestinal villi in the celiac child will be club-shaped and may be shorter than normal. Villi are also markedly fewer in number than normal, providing a decreased ability to hydrolyze gluten. Studies have shown that exacerbations and remissions are common in this disorder. Furthermore, if left untreated, lactose intolerance will result as secondary to the destruction of the intestinal villi. Therefore, children with celiac disease who are not in remission will need to be on a milk-free diet in addition to being on a gluten-free diet. Later, when the disease is under control and the villi have repaired themselves, milk may be reintroduced.

The treatment for celiac disease is strictly dietary. First, the child must be placed on a gluten-free and milk-free diet. Then, because malabsorption of other nutrients often occurs, the child needs a good assessment of his or her nutritional status, and a diet providing all the proper nutrients is introduced. For some children this may mean taking iron supplements or vitamin D supplements. A good working relationship with the child's physician and a registered dietitian will be very beneficial.

Gluten is a vegetable protein. It is present in wheat, rye, barley, buckwheat, and oats. It is also present in rice and potatoes, although studies have shown that these two foods do not evoke symptoms in the celiac child. Children who must eat a gluten-free diet have a very difficult challenge ahead of them, and the diet often takes several weeks to show any positive effect. This is due to the time necessary for the intestinal mucosa to repair itself and for the secondary lactose intolerance to subside.

After a period of usually two years, a gluten challenge test may be given and an intestinal biopsy may be performed to check the status of the intestinal villi. At this point, most children with confirmed celiac disease probably will not outgrow the problem. Many adults today who have digestive distress are now tested and treated for celiac disease, and the problem is thought to be more prevalent than previously reported.

RAP—Recurrent Abdominal Pain

Infants and children have suffered tummy aches since the beginning of time. Figuring out exactly what is causing the problem is tricky, even for pediatricians, who treat infants and children day after day. Recurrent abdominal pain, or RAP, is so common in infants and children, it could be classified as a therapeutic nightmare. Abdominal pain is a constituent of so many diseases and medical situations from stress and fear to flu and urinary tract infection.

Babies with recurrent abdominal pain are sometimes dismissed as colicky—parents are told the pain is just the result of their being infants. Often the only advice parents are given by pediatricians is that there is nothing to do but live with it. However there have been a limited number of studies that link infant colic or recurrent abdominal pain to a sensitivity to cow's milk formula. Experts in the field of lactose intolerance and milk allergy often advise the trial elimination of cow's milk formula or cow's milk from the diet of a breast-feeding mother as a test to determine whether or not the elimination or reduction of cow's milk in the diet improves the reported abdominal pain in infants.

During the 1970s, studies were done on young children who had frequent tummy aches (as often as once a month for several months in a row). Scientists learned that as many as 15 percent of children who see pediatricians suffer with pain in the abdomen this frequently. The syndrome seems to begin after age four and peaks between six and seven years of age. Some of the common factors seen in children with RAP are pallor, headache, constipation, a history of colic as infants, and an interruption of daily activities due to abdominal pain. Twenty-eight percent of the children studied were absent from school more than one day in ten. Some of the children studied actually had peptic ulcers. A few had urinary tract infections, but the absence of organic disease was most common. Follow-up studies showed that very rarely some of these children grew up to develop inflammatory bowel disease.

Most children with RAP do not have any organic disease, but fully 40 percent of them are deficient in the lactase enzyme, although they do not exhibit many of the common symptoms of lactose intolerance and therefore do not receive correct testing and diagnosis. According to John B. Watkins, M.D., chief of gastroenterology and nutrition, Children's Hospital of Philadelphia, and associate professor of pediatrics, University of Pennsylvania, "Physicians have difficulty in diagnosing recurrent abdominal pain and excluding organic disease." Dr. Watkins explains his conclusion after reviewing a 1978 study by Liebman of 119 youngsters who were subjected to a large number of diagnostic tests before their physicians were comfortable with a nonorganic diagnosis. Of the 119 children in the study, 99 had upper gastrointestinal series; 52 had barium enemas; 34 had intravenous pyelograms; 22 had fiber optic endoscopy; and 18 had proctoscopy and rectal biopsy. Some received upper endoscopy or exploratory laparotomy. Dr. Watkins explains that these tests were routinely done, "despite strong evidence that such procedures are futile."

Experts in the field then looked to primary lactose intolerance as a cause of recurrent abdominal pain in children. Albert

Newcomer, M.D., professor of medicine, Division of Gastro-enterology and Internal Medicine, Mayo Clinic, Rochester, Minnesota, and Jack D. Welsh, M.D., professor of medicine, University of Oklahoma in Oklahoma City, conducted studies in 1977 and 1978 that showed that the decline in lactase enzyme activity may often take place somewhat earlier than popularly thought, without mucosal damage or acute diarrhea. In other words, lactose intolerance may be operating in children who do not present with diarrhea or other symptoms of malabsorption. These children chiefly complain of pain in their tummy. Studies done of recurrent abdominal pain conducted by Dr. Theodore Bayless and others during the 1970s and 1980s confirmed that lactose intolerance was prevalent in children with RAP and that symptomatic evidence proved to be an unreliable means of diagnosing lactose intolerance in children with RAP.

Over and over, parents are told that their children who suffer with tummy aches do so as a result of psychological stresses. This attitude is reinforced when physicians do clinical tests to determine organic causes of recurrent abdominal pain, and none are found. The expert information, however, indicates that lactose intolerance should be suspected from the onset, and that a milk-free diet should be tried before concluding that the child has a psychological problem.

Colic

In book after book, parents can read that infantile colic has no known cause or cure. The periodic wailing of a baby who seems to be overcome with abdominal pain, sometimes for hours at a time, is often dismissed by pediatricians or attributed to the inexperience of mothers and fathers. A range of explanations for colic have been offered, from excess stimulation to feeding incompetence. But some recent, excellent scientific studies about infant colic have shown a potential relationship between infant colic and milk. While not necessarily always conclusive, this information may be helpful to parents coping with a colicky baby.

In April 1991, as reported in the American Academy of Pediatrics journal *Pediatrics,* Patrick S. Clyne, M.D., and Anthony Kulczycki, M.D., published findings that suggest that certain antibodies produced by cows contribute to colic in susceptible infants. While previous studies have shown that unidentified proteins in cow's milk might cause colic in some infants, even infants fed breast milk exclusively, the Clyne-Kulczycki study has pinpointed a specific type of cow's protein associated with colic, namely, antibodies called immunoglobulin G (IgG).

The researchers looked for IgG in milk from fifty-nine nursing mothers and found that the concentrations averaged 31 percent higher in mothers with colicky babies than in those with noncolicky babies. Incredibly, they also discovered that 86 percent of the women, including those with noncolicky babies, showed bovine IgG concentrations at least two hundred times higher than the levels of the other bovine proteins measured in earlier studies. This indicates that women who are nursing colicky babies should pay close attention to the amount of cow's milk protein they ingest because the IgG antibodies are passed through the breast milk. The mothers were advised to give up dairy products for at least a week to see if their baby's colic improved and, at the same time, to maintain their calcium levels with supplements.

In October 1989, in the same journal, Dr. Al Kahn of the Pediatric Sleep Unit at University Children's Hospital, Free University of Brussels, and the University Clinic Ersame conducted a study of seventeen infants who had persistent sleep disturbances. These infants did not respond to conventional therapy, and Dr. Kahn wanted to test the theory of milk sensitivity and its negative correlation to sleep. All the infants in the study had milk totally withdrawn from their diet. The results were striking: fifteen of the seventeen infants fell asleep faster, had far fewer waking episodes, and their total sleep time per 24 hours increased from an average of 5.5 hours to 13 hours. In order to test the theory beyond reproach, Dr. Kahn then challenged these same infants with cow's milk. All of the improved infants developed sleep disturbances again, and these disturbances disappeared when cow's milk was withdrawn from the diet a second time, proving conclusively that milk sensitivity may have a profound effect on sleep for some infants.

Crohn's Disease

Inflammatory bowel disease (IBD) is a term used to describe several different conditions that affect approximately two million Americans. In fact, it is estimated that about 200,000 children are afflicted with one or more of the IBDs, which include Crohn's disease and ulcerative colitis. Crohn's disease typically strikes young people between the ages of fifteen and thirty, commonly presenting during the eighteen- to twenty-five-year range. The cause of Crohn's disease is as yet unknown, and there is no cure. To be sure, having Crohn's is like riding a roller coaster of remission and relapse, often throughout one's adult life. Symptoms of Crohn's include diarrhea and cramping, often with intense pain on the right side. The patient usually has a low-grade fever and complains of feeling generally ill.

Because these symptoms may occur undramatically or may be mistaken for a transitory flu, many young people with Crohn's remain undiagnosed for a long time. The diagnosis is confirmed after a variety of clinical tests are done, usually including blood tests, stool analyses, and radiographic and/or endoscopic procedures. Crohn's leaves a definite mark on the inside of the intestine, which is detectable by the trained eye.

The problem in Crohn's disease is a chronic inflammation of the intestinal tract, most often involving the ileum and colon (both the small and large intestine). Acute attacks may force a hospital stay and, under some circumstances, the disease may be life threatening. There can also be inflammation elsewhere, including the ankles, knees, wrists, or other joints. Patients with Crohn's may have mouth sores, inflammation in the eyes, or tender nodules over the lower leg. Malabsorption and malnutrition typically occur due to the fact that inflammation occurs in precisely the areas of the digestive system that house the digestive enzymes.

The treatment for Crohn's includes cortisone (steroids) to fight the inflammation, given either by mouth, injection, intravenously, or through an enema. Other anti-inflammatory drugs may also be used. Surgery is sometimes attempted with Crohn's, but is most likely used to relieve specific complications of the disease such as abscesses, fistulas, or strictures.

Children and young adults with active Crohn's, which involves inflammation and diarrhea, will experience a depletion of the lactase enzyme as a secondary condition. For this reason, dairy foods should be eliminated during an attack of Crohn's. Otherwise, no special diet is universally recommended. But it is very important that parents help see to it that their child with Crohn's is fed properly, especially during an inflammatory period. Good nutrition is essential to replace the vitamins and minerals lost due to the malabsorption caused by inflammation. The maintenance of a dairy-free diet is also necessary to prevent further damage to the intestinal villi during the time when the disease is active. Milk and other dairy foods may be reintroduced during periods of remission.

There is an emotional component to Crohn's disease that cannot be ignored, especially when dealing with young children and highly sensitive teenagers. Kids need the strong support of their parents and friends at this time, particularly if they are in the hospital. Also it is important to realize that kids may feel embarrassed by the nature of their disease. If this is a problem, parents should be sensitive enough not to discuss the details of the disease or treatment with their child's friends. There may be other facets to Crohn's that children have difficulty coping with including physical pain, self-pity, and self-consciousness. Counseling is available through a variety of organizations that serve to support families dealing with Crohn's, and professional counseling has proven to be invaluable to families coping with the disease.

Ulcerative Colitis

Ulcerative colitis is another of the IBDs, or inflammatory bowel diseases, that typically strike teenagers or young adults. It involves a diffuse inflammation and ulcerative disease of the large intestine and often looks strikingly similar to Crohn's disease. Bloody diarrhea and pain plague the ulcerative colitis patient, who will also present with dehydration, weight loss, fever, anemia, and general debility.

Children with ulcerative colitis require special attention. Their diet must be strong in nutrients. But there is an emotional as well as a physical component to consider. These children will need support, education, and love. Professional counseling can be extremely beneficial to families coping with ulcerative colitis. Treatment for the disease usually includes anti-inflammatory medication, surgery, and individualized dietary plans. Usually very low residue diets are begun at first and then altered depending upon the patient's physical response. As in Crohn's disease, secondary lactose intolerance will be present, and the proper dairy-restricted diet must be followed.

Cystic Fibrosis

Cystic fibrosis is a disease that afflicts infants, children, and young adults. It is an autosomal recessive disorder, meaning that it is hereditary and both parents must carry the recessive gene in order for their child to inherit the disease. Cystic fibro-

sis is a very serious disease, incurable so far, although much research is underway that has brought important information to
the medical community, not the least of which is the identification of the specific gene location. More research is still needed
in order to find a cure, but generally, children with CF are living longer and healthier lives today than their counterparts
even fifteen years ago.

Cystic fibrosis is characterized by a dysfunction of the ex-
ocrine glands (glands that discharge secretions through ducts)
involving abnormal levels of mucus secretion, which obstruct
ducts in the pancreas, lungs, liver, and intestine. Because of pan-
creatic involvement, essential enzymes are not released, seriously
interfering with the digestion of proteins, fats, and carbohydrates. Diarrhea is common and respiratory involvement is a
hallmark of CF. Infants and children have chronic pulmonary
disease and bronchial obstruction, usually requiring daily treatments aimed at dislodging bronchial mucus buildup.

Children with CF take various enzymes in chewable form
before eating. Often, as much as half of the protein and fat in
their diet goes undigested. For many children, the orally administered enzymes help prevent that nutritional loss. Children with
severe intestinal involvement will not be able to tolerate any
dairy products. Others may suffer from varying degrees of lactose intolerance. The use of lactase enzyme supplements is
prevalent in treating CF, although dairy intake usually has to be
quite restricted.

Abnormally high levels of sodium and chloride—up to two
and a half times normal—are found in the sweat of CF babies
and children. In fact, measurement of sweat chloride is often the
first step in the diagnosis of the disease. Parents of infants with
frequently occurring diarrhea often can taste the excess sodium
in their baby's sweat by kissing the child. Any infant who tastes
salty should be referred to his or her pediatrician for further testing. Other symptoms of cystic fibrosis include lethargy, weight
loss, and failure to thrive.

Galactosemia

Galactosemia is a congenital birth defect classified as an "inborn error of metabolism." It is caused by the absence or abnormality of one of the enzymes required to convert galactose to glucose. Galactose is absorbed, but builds up in the blood and tissues. Soon after birth, infants unable to completely hydrolyze galactose present with symptoms of vomiting, diarrhea, lethargy, jaundice, and puffiness of the face and lower extremities. There may be an enlarged spleen, liver damage, and cataracts. The infant with galactosemia fails to gain weight and soon becomes malnourished. If left untreated, galactosemia may cause brain damage and death. However, when properly treated after early detection through urinalysis and blood tests, children born with galactosemia may not suffer dread reactions and are likely to have minimal if any damage to the brain. When treatment is instituted, the symptoms caused by the galactosemia generally abate.

Galactose is present only in a very limited number of foods. Milk is the most common source. Lactose, the carbohydrate in milk, is composed of glucose and galactose. Therefore, babies born with the inability to hydrolyze galactose must be treated with milk-free diets and placed on appropriate formulas. Soy formulas are not always substituted due to the theory that a component of the carbohydrate in soybeans is hydrolyzed to galactose. This has not been proven definitively, although it is common practice to restrict the child's intake of soybeans, beets, lima beans, and peas, which all contain the suspect carbohydrate stachyose. Other foods that contain galactose are organ meats such as liver, pancreas, and brains.

Mothers of infants with galactosemia may themselves have diminished ability to digest galactose, although galactosemia per se may be undiagnosed. If a mother with limited ability to digest galactose drinks extremely large amounts of milk during her pregnancy, and her child inherits the galactosemia, the fetus may be irreparably damaged due to the fact that galactose passes through the placenta. Families with a history of this disease require genetic counseling in order to learn how to cope with potentially affected children. Galactosemia is detectable through amniocentesis, which helps parents determine for certain whether or not their unborn child has the disease, and if so, treatment consisting of a milk-free diet for the mother may begin early in an attempt to stave off future difficulties for the baby.

Surgery, Cancer, and AIDS

Thankfully, most children in this country are generally healthy and are able to eat a diverse diet made up of all kinds of foods available. Rarely, however, some children are subjected to surgical removal of areas of their digestive system due to disease or blockages. This surgery renders them unable to properly metabolize some foods, including milk and other dairy products. Similarly, children subjected to radiation therapy or chemotherapy for malignancies will have their digestive systems negatively affected and require milk-free diets in most cases. The same is true for children with immune system diseases such as AIDS who will be unable to digest cow's milk due to an inability to hydrolyze the protein in milk. Children with liver disease, who must restrict their intake of protein, are usually placed on dairy-restricted diets due to the large portion of protein in a milk serving. Children who must cope with unusual medical conditions such as cancer, surgery, or AIDS are often treated with digestive enzymes or other alternative feeding regimens, including prehydrolyzed infant formulas.

Wherever your child fits in this discussion of medical conditions, be assured that alternatives to milk and other dairy foods are easily available and will give your child all the nutritional components he or she needs to grow. As you will learn, milk is not the only source of calcium. Milk is not the only source of vitamin D. And milk is not the only source of phosphorus, magnesium, or protein—far from it. Your child, no matter what his or her medical condition, need not be denied any of the nutrients needed to grow simply because he or she cannot consume milk. Soon, you will learn where to find the essential nutritional elements you are looking for and how to widen your child's food horizons.

2 The Dairy-Free Diet Merry-Go-Round

When kids think of being on a merry-go-round, they probably think of the fun they have picking out the one special painted horse that bids them to climb up, or the joy they have spinning on that beautifully painted horse as the wind blows across their cheeks and through their hair while they hum along with the unmistakable music of the carousel. But to adults the expression "being on a merry-go-round" does not evoke the same kind of positive feeling that it does for children. "Being on a merry-go-round" can also imply the negative experience one has when searching for answers that are difficult to find or trying to come up with solutions, only to be given conflicting or inaccurate information that makes the problem more convoluted, rather than more understandable.

Parents who are confronted with the responsibility of altering their child's diet in such a major way as reducing or eliminating milk and other dairy foods may feel like they are indeed on a merry-go-round. First, sources of information are very limited. Not many books have been written about this issue. In fact, only four or five books have been published in the last fifteen years or so that are dedicated to a dairy-free lifestyle. Second, many health-care givers are not well versed in the daily management of lactose intolerance or milk allergy and can therefore offer only minimal help to parents coping with this dietary restriction. Often, parents are given a sheet that lists some foods to eat and some foods to avoid and little else. The advice may be simple enough ("If it bothers you, don't eat it"), but it is hardly comprehensive. Usually the help of a registered dietitian is not initiated through the physician's office, and this is unfortunate. In fact, of the thousands of people who have read my books or subscribed to my newsletter and have written to me to share their experiences, only a tiny fraction were ever referred to a professional for help with dietary management. Mostly, parents are left to cope as best they can, with very little support and very little reliable information available to answer their questions and address their concerns about their child's health.

The most critical question parents have right from the start is, of course, "What will I feed my child today?" This is a question that is often responded to with what sounds like an easy answer: "Nothing with milk in it." But because milk and its by-products are so pervasive in our food, the answer is bound to be more complicated than it sounds. So, what I propose here, is to reconfigure our perception of the merry-go-round to give it a new meaning, one that is helpful to parents of dairy-sensitive children. In an effort to make the metaphor work, imagine a "dairy-free diet merry-go-round" composed of beautiful and healthful horses, each one representing a specific food category from which to make selections every day for your child. This variety of choices will be the foundation of your child's individualized dairy-free diet. You and your child will pick and choose foods that are appealing, nutritious, and taste great.

Basic Food Choices

The following food categories represent the painted horses on our dairy-free diet merry-go-round. A little understanding of the nutrients in these foods compared to those in milk will help you make good choices in the formulation of a balanced and healthy dairy-free diet for your child. A more complete dairy-free diet list follows this section.

Fruits, Vegetables, and Legumes

No food that is harvested from the ground contains milk. Milk comes from mammary glands, which are present only in mammals. Plants do not have any mammary glands and therefore contain no milk protein, no milk sugar (lactose), in fact, no milk in any form. So the first element of the dairy-free diet must be plant food. *All fruits, vegetables, and legumes may be included in the diet of the lactose-intolerant or milk-allergic child.*

Some fruits, vegetables and legumes are preferred choices in a dairy-free diet, based on their calcium content. Excellent vegetable choices are the dark green, leafy ones such as broccoli and other greens such as kale, turnip, and mustard. Another vegetable high in calcium content is bok choy (chinese cabbage). Legumes are beans, peas, and nuts; several varieties of legumes have a high calcium content, including black beans, garbanzo beans, and navy beans. Many fruits contain calcium, although generally the mineral content is low. However, there are some bright stars in this category such as dried apricots, dates, dried peaches, raisins, and blackberries.

Some fruits, vegetables, and legumes may appear on a "high calcium" list but are not actually desirable as mineral sources. This is because some of these, while high in calcium content, also contain oxalic acid, a substance that interferes with the absorption of calcium and actually may deplete calcium stores if eaten in very large amounts. Fruits and vegetables containing oxalic acid include cranberries, rhubarb, chard, gooseberries, and spinach. In the legume family, nuts such as almonds, walnuts, and sesame seeds may be high in calcium, but also contain oxalates.

The only real exceptions to the axiom that "all fruits, vegetables, and legumes may be included in the diet of the lactose-intolerant or milk-allergic child," come from the fact that some fruits and vegetables in the marketplace are processed into canned, frozen, or otherwise packaged dishes that have added milk, milk protein, or lactose. Many frozen vegetables, for instance, are packaged with accompanying sauces or gravies that contain casein or whey. Some frozen fruits may have added sugar syrups, some of which include lactose. If the fruits or vegetables you select are not fresh, it is imperative that you read all labels and make your selections accordingly.

Meats, Fish, and Poultry

A variety of meats, fish, and poultry are available to the lactose-intolerant or milk-allergic child. Again, because animals from the sea (with the exception of a few, such as dolphins or whales) are not mammals, they are completely free of milk. The same is true of poultry including chicken, turkey, duck, goose, and others. Beef, lamb, veal, and venison are certainly acceptable food choices on a dairy-free diet, although these animals are mammals and do nurse their young. There has been some anecdotal evidence to suggest that occasionally children who are allergic to the protein in animal milk may react to eating the flesh of that animal as well, particularly beef. Therefore, when dealing with a highly allergic child, it may be best to avoid beef and stick to fish and poultry at first.

Meats, fish, and poultry are rich in a variety of nutrients that will encourage your child's growth and good health. Some of the most important for your child include protein, the B vitamins, vitamin A, and iron. Some fish do have a relatively substantial calcium content because their bones, which house their calcium stores, are so small and soft that they may be eaten. The best to choose are sardines, canned salmon, and canned mackerel.

Eggs and Peanut Butter

While these two foods have probably never been lumped together in any official nutritional analysis or food group, they may very well play an exceedingly important role in your child's dairy-free diet. The reason is simple: Many children love eggs and peanut butter, although not necessarily served together. As far as nutrients go, these two are terrific foods. While one is from an animal source and the other from a plant source, they are comparable sources of protein in the diet. One egg has about the same amount of protein as two tablespoons of peanut butter. The peanut butter contains about 18 mg of calcium and the egg about 25. The egg also contains about 590 IU of vitamin A, 129 mg potassium, 205 mg phosphorus, 11 mg magnesium, and 5 μg of folic acid, an essential nutrient for growth. Peanut butter contains 202 mg of potassium, 136 mg phosphorus, 58 mg magnesium, and 20 μg folic acid. It is also rich in vitamin B_6.

While many parents are concerned about the fat or cholesterol content of these two foods, it is very important to note several things with regard to feeding children. First, an abundance of fatty foods in the diet does not make sense for anyone, children or adults. But some fats are essential, healthful, and protective, and children do require fat in their diet for proper growth and health. One egg contains two grams of saturated fat, about the same amount as in one cup of yogurt made from skim milk, and three grams of unsaturated fat. Eggs also provide the most complete protein available. Two tablespoons of peanut butter contain four grams of saturated fat, a bit more than one cup of 2-percent milk, which contains about three grams of saturated fat, and twelve grams of unsaturated fat.

The unsaturated fats such as those found in peanut butter and eggs are the fats of choice when selecting foods appropriate for your child. These so-called "good" fats do not contribute to the formation of plaque in the arteries.

Many people avoid eggs because of concerns about cholesterol. But even adults who are limiting their cholesterol intake from food are able to eat four to six eggs per week, and cholesterol is usually not an issue for children (unless they have a very unusual medical condition that might require the limitation of cholesterol from food sources). But remember that the three main food categories that provide cholesterol in the diet are dairy products, red meat, and eggs. Your child will not be eating dairy products, or at least not substantial amounts of dairy products and you can limit your child's intake of red meat if you choose. Feel free to let your child enjoy eggs.

When compared to other typical kinds of foods kids enjoy eating, eggs and peanut butter come out way ahead of some of the other very popular choices. For example, there are about five grams of fat in one egg, half saturated, and half unsaturated, compared to about seventeen grams of fat in a hamburger. In one tablespoon of peanut butter, you will find about eight grams of fat, only two grams saturated, and the other six grams unsaturated, compared to fifteen grams of fat in one hot dog, all of it saturated. This information suggests that eggs and peanut butter should be favorably accepted by conscientious parents as excellent choices of high-protein foods for their children. And the best part is that both of these foods are totally milk-free.

Grain Products

Grains, in and of themselves, are all milk-free. Grain products are now considered to be the backbone of a healthy diet for all children and adults. By current nutrition standards, today's children are advised to eat about nine servings from the grain group each day. These may include breads, pastas, rice, or cereal. A complete discussion of the new food group recommendations is included in this chapter.

Unless the diagnosis is celiac disease, grains served simply are all right for lactose-intolerant or milk-allergic children to eat. For the most part, dairy-sensitive children can have plain pasta of all sorts, rice of all varieties, oats, barley, wheat germ, quinoa, and more. Prepared breads and cereals present a bit of a challenge, though, because milk is sometimes added to these products during baking or processing. However, most "ethnic" types of breads are milk-free, including authentic French, Italian, pita, bagels, and rye. Corn and flour tortillas are also milk-free. The typically American sorts of white breads and rolls based on old farm recipes are often made with milk, scalded milk, or buttermilk. While baking may cause some molecular changes in the milk, these white breads still may not be well tolerated by either the lactose-intolerant or milk-allergic child.

Many prepared cold cereals are milk-free and may be eaten as snacks or for meals. These cereals may be served with a milk-substitute or sprinkled on top of cut-up fruit or dairy-free

ice creams or casseroles. Often they are fortified with extra vitamins and minerals and will make a solid contribution to your
child's dairy-free diet. Likewise, many warm cereals are available
to your child such as oatmeal and Cream of Wheat. While many
people like to top these warm cereals with milk, it is certainly
not a requirement. To enhance their flavor, they may be topped
with a dollop of jam or milk-free margarine. Again, parents
must be aware of overprocessed packaged hot cereal products.
Many flavored hot cereals contain milk or milk by-products. The
information should be on the ingredient label, although sometimes this information isn't clear. Later in this chapter you will
learn exactly how to read a food label and will discover precisely
which added ingredients mean milk even when the word "milk"
isn't spelled out.

Treats and Junque Food

Unfortunately, not all parents and children are perfect. They all
indulge in a little "junque" periodically. So, let's not try to pre-
tend that our children will not be fed treats. Instead let's make
sure that when they do eat foods that are somewhat to the left of
the four food groups, at least those foods are not laden with
milk. They may not be the most healthful choices to include in
your child's diet, but treats, snacks, baked goods, and candy are
bound to show up in the dairy-free diet merry-go-round, invited
or not. So be prepared to make the best of it.

Cakes, cookies, muffins, and other baked goods are, in general, all made with milk, unless they are baked at home using
milk-free recipes, purchased in a store or kosher bakery as parve
items (this will be explained shortly), or belong to a particular
group of baked goods that are called "air cakes." Air cakes include sponge cake, angel food cake, and usually jelly roll. Cakes
that contain a substantial amount of fruit, such as apple cake or
banana cake, are often milk-free because the liquid and sugar in
the fruit serves to create molecular changes during the baking
process that are similar to those created by milk. Some cookies

that are traditionally milk-free include snickerdoodles and oat-meal cookies. Of course, recipes may differ, and it is always wise to check ingredients when possible.

Many crunchy treats are also milk-free. These include pretzels, regular potato chips, potato sticks, plain tortilla chips, and plain popcorn. Rice cakes are milk-free and now come in a variety of treatlike flavors for snacks. Another very popular treat that is milk-free is the baked cereal/pretzel/peanut mixture often made with the Chex cereals. Some of the packaged varieties do contain cheese chips, but this is a treat that is easily made at home as a dairy-free recipe.

There are a variety of milk-free "ice creams" available today. Some are made from lactose-reduced milk, some are based on soy products, some are based on rice, some are based on fruit. Some familiar brand names include Rice Dream, Tofutti, This Is Blis, and Mocha Mix. There are several frozen fruit treats on the market including Popsicles, Dole Fruit 'n' Juice Bars, and some sorbets.

Candy is a treat that most all children love, and many kinds of candy are milk-free, including many chocolates. Hard candies and lollipops are almost always milk-free. So are the fruity gooey candies such as Starburst, Gummy Bears, jelly beans, and licorice. Chocolate may contain milk and may not. All milk chocolate contains milk. Some dark or semisweet chocolates may contain milk, but some varieties do not. Often chocolate-covered mint candy such as Junior Mints is milk-free. Certainly chocolate confections made at home from pure baking chocolate or cocoa powder or plain chocolate syrup, none of which contain milk, are permissible. A more detailed discussion of chocolate is found later in this chapter.

Beverages

Many beverages are milk-free and may be enjoyed by your child, including fruit drinks such as lemonade, limeade, fruit coolers, and juices. The very popular athletic thirst quenchers are milk-free, as are fruit drink mixes. These drinks may be blended with pieces of fruit and ice for a more nutritious and rich special drink that kids will love. Of course colas and other soda pops are milk-free as are coffee and tea.

One interesting beverage item that parents might want to include in their child's diet is mineral water. Many of these naturally carbonated waters are rich in calcium and can provide an additional calcium source in your child's diet. Mineral water may be flavored, blended, or used in cooking. Some of the brands that contain the highest amounts of calcium are Contrexeville, Ferrarelle, and Mendocino.

Tofu

A relatively new food in the American diet is tofu, the curd made from soybean "milk." Tofu, long a staple in the Asian diet, is an interesting food that can be utilized in so many ways that there is bound to be one your child will enjoy. Tofu is often called "soy cheese" because it is made by a process similar to the manufacture of cow's milk cheese. The soybeans are cooked, and the liquid is then separated from the product. What remains is tofu, a soft or semisoft cheesy-looking product that has a very mild taste.

Tofu can be eaten plain, sliced for a sandwich, cubed and tossed into soups or casseroles, breaded and fried, or sautéed with other vegetables in a stir-fry. What makes tofu so special, however, is that it is milk-free, low in fat, cholesterol free, and it contains about 150 mg of calcium in a four-ounce serving. When blended with fresh or frozen fruit, it looks, tastes, and feels like yogurt, but has no dairy component whatsoever. This is a food you may want to experiment with if you are unfamiliar with it, but please make room for this choice in your child's dairy-free diet.

Calcium-Enriched Products

Because of recent scientific research about calcium in the American diet, food manufacturers have been producing a variety of calcium-fortified products. Recent research indicates several things about calcium in the American diet. First, its importance is notably earned as calcium has proven to be a component of high blood pressure, osteoporosis, and cancer. Second, researchers have learned that as a group, Americans probably eat only one- to two-thirds the amount of calcium required each day. And worse, as people shift from high-fat diets to low-fat diets, with the elimination of fatty dairy foods, experts believe that the calcium intake of Americans will plummet further. Third, Americans receive very mixed messages regarding vitamin supplementation. We are told that in a typical American diet, supplementation should not be necessary because our food can provide all the nutrients needed. But because most Americans do not avail themselves of the wide scope of healthful foods in the marketplace, we are often vitamin and mineral deficient, and probably need, but do not take, supplements. A diet of hot dogs and chips will simply not cut it.

So, in response to recent nutritional findings, the recognition of lactose intolerance and milk allergy, and consumer demand, food manufacturers have been cooking up all sorts of ways to sneak extra calcium into food that normally contains none. Many of these foods will be a boon to your child's dairy-free diet. They include a variety calcium-fortified juices; some calcium-fortified cereals, perfect for snacking; and calcium-fortified breads. While, in reality, there is virtually no difference between a child taking a calcium supplement or eating calcium-enriched foods, often it will be easier to accomplish supplemation through food rather than through another form.

Milk Substitutes

Instead of cow's milk, there are literally scores of milklike substitutes in the marketplace. These substitutes may be used in place of milk for many recipes, including some baking recipes, although a little experimentation may be necessary to achieve just the right result. After all, baking is a chemical process that requires just the right proportion of heat, sugar, leavening agents, liquids, and more. Milk, because it contains liquid and sugar, may be difficult to replace exactly in baked recipes, but that does not mean it is irreplaceable. Your favorite recipes can be made with soy milks, or dairy-free creamers, or casein-based milks, if your child is not allergic to them. Often in a recipe, the milk may be replaced by applesauce or mashed banana or orange juice— all foods with a high liquid and sugar content.

The same is true of milk-free infant formula. While it may not taste fabulous to the connoisseur, diluted formula may work very well in a zucchini muffin recipe or to dilute condensed soup. It is certainly acceptable to the baby who has grown up on it and may make a great topping for oatmeal or dry cereal.

Basically, milk substitutes fall into the following categories and are used best in the following manner:

Fruit juice   Useful in the making of pancakes, waffles, french toast, egg washes, gravies, and sauces. It is acceptable for children with lactose intolerance or milk allergy.

Soy milk   A nutty flavored product that works well in many recipes and as an accompaniment to hot or cold cereal. It is acceptable for children with lactose intolerance or milk allergy. Some children, however, are allergic to soy protein and should therefore not use soy products.

Casein milk   A variety of these have shown up in the marketplace recently. Some, such as Vitamite, are decades old, but have been re-dressed for the nineties. These milk substitutes work well in almost all hot or cold applications, but are not appropriate for children with milk allergy, due to the fact that casein is a milk protein. However, they may work wonderfully in the diet of the lactose-intolerant child.

Nondairy creamers   Several of these products are offered by Rich Products, Carnation, and Mocha Mix, and a multitude of locally produced brands may be found in supermarkets. Nondairy creamers are not ideal nutritionally because some of them contain saturated fats, but they may be used occasionally in recipes calling for small quantities of milk. Rich Products also manufactures a product called Richwhip that is available as a completely dairy-free ready-to-whip frozen product or as a lactose-free nondairy prepared whipped topping. The former product is perfect for making milk-free ice cream or whipped-cream toppings and mousses. The latter product is useful for children who are not allergic to milk protein and is used as you would use other whipped toppings. Many of the nondairy creamer products contain whey and/or casein and may not be acceptable for either lactose-intolerant or milk-allergic children. Label reading is essential.

Infant formulas   These are ideal for babies and toddlers who require lots of calories, vitamins, and minerals. There are soy-milk formulas containing no dairy products whatsoever; prehydrolyzed formulas, which are cow's milk based, but all the lactose and all the milk proteins have been predigested; and there are lactose-free milk-based formulas. A complete discussion of infant formulas occurs in Chapter 4. These products may be used in cooking and, when diluted, as beverages long after infancy. Obviously lactose-free formulas will be acceptable for lactose-intolerant children, soy-milk formulas will be acceptable for either lactose-intolerant or milk-protein allergic children, and prehydrolyzed formulas should be acceptable to either child.

Lactase enzyme-treated milks   The only true way to decrease or eliminate lactose from the milk is to treat it with a lactase enzyme causing hydrolysis to occur. Enzyme-treated milks vary in their lactose content. Some milks have the lactose eliminated by 70 percent, others claim between 90 percent and 100 percent lactose hydrolysis. The enzymes which do the work best are derived from the fungal agent *Aspergillus niger* or the enzyme beta-galactosidase.

Some familiar brand names of enzyme treated milk include Lactaid and Dairy Ease. A number of more localized manufacturers, such as Dean and Kemp's and others, manufacture enzyme-treated milk. Check the local dairies in your area for more information. You may also treat milk with enzymes in your own kitchen and will learn exactly how to do this later in the book.

Enzyme-treated milks are used in the manufacture of lactose-reduced cheese or ice cream. Some of the more familiar brand names of lactose-reduced or lactose-free cheeses are Soymage and Formagg, Smart Beat, and Lactaid. These products may not be suitable for children with milk-protein allergy because lactase enzymes do not affect proteins at all.

Planning the Diet

There are three basic dairy-free diets. One eliminates all sources of lactose. This is appropriate for the lactose-intolerant child who needs to watch out only for milk sugar. Another dairy-free diet eliminates all sources of milk protein. This diet is appropriate for the child with a milk allergy who develops immune-system symptoms after ingesting milk. This child may be able to tolerate lactose, but will react to the protein component in milk.

The third and most inclusive dairy-free diet is the one that eliminates all sources of lactose and milk protein. This diet is most appropriate when it has not been determined precisely which condition the child has or when the child may in fact be both lactose intolerant and allergic to milk protein. This diet may also be the best one for all children prone to frequent digestive upsets, regardless of the cause. It's certainly the safest bet for children sensitive to milk and the one recommended to start with when beginning to construct an individualized dairy-free diet for your child.

Milk-Free Foods to Enjoy

Angel food cake

Bagels

Baking chocolate

Bread stuffing/dressing

Broth

Clear soups

Cocoa powder

Colas/soda pop

Condiments/mayonnaise/
mustard/ketchup

Cream of Wheat

Eggs

Ethnic breads/breadsticks

Fish

French/Italian bread

Fruit drinks

Fruits

Gelatin

Hard candies

Jams/jellies/preserves

Legumes

Lemonade/limeade

Licorice

Marshmallows

Meats

Mineral water

Nuts

Oatmeal

Olives

Pasta

Pickles

Pita bread

Popcorn

Potato chips

Poultry

Pretzels

Rice

Soy products

Sponge cake

Tofu

Tortillas (corn and flour)

Vegetables

Wheat germ

Eliminating Lactose

Lactose, as you now know, is the sugar or carbohydrate in milk. It is a component of *all milk*. I frequently tell readers, when they ask me if a certain milk is okay for them to have, to remember that if it *says* milk, it *is* milk, and all milk derived from animals contains lactose. This includes goat's milk, cow's milk, and buffalo milk. It includes acidophilus milk, lactose-reduced milk, skim milk, and powdered milk. The only milks that do *not* contain lactose are soy milk and some artificial milks made from the milk protein casein. Even milks that claim to have the lactose reduced by 100 percent may *still* contain small amounts of lactose, as our current labeling regulations do allow for "insignificant" amounts of lactose to be left in enzyme-treated milk products. So, if you want to eliminate all sources of lactose from food, you will want to eliminate all milk.

This includes all other dairy products made from milk such as cheese, yogurt, and ice cream. While it is possible that your child may be able to tolerate milk or cheese or yogurt to some degree, it is best to eliminate all sources of lactose in the diet of the lactose-intolerant child when beginning the process of developing a proper diet regimen. Later, in Chapter 4 you will learn how to ascertain your child's tolerance level for lactose and may then adjust his or her diet accordingly (see Table 2.1).

As far as additives are concerned, there are two that appear on ingredient labels and must be avoided. They are *lactose* and *whey*. Lactose is, of course, the offending sugar, and whey is the liquid portion of the milk that is drawn off during cheese making. Because lactose is water soluble, it travels with the whey during the separation process. It does not matter whether or not the whey is used in its liquid form or in its dried form. It still contains lactose.

Eliminating Milk Protein

Milk protein is a component of all milk. It is in all types of milk, cheese, ice cream, and yogurt. Therefore, all forms of milk and dairy foods must be avoided by the milk-allergic child. Again, each allergic child will have his or her own threshold of tolerance at which point he or she will negatively react to allergens such as cow's milk protein. Determining the allergic threshold will be discussed in Chapter 4, but for our initial purposes it is

Table 2.1 Lactose Content of Dairy Foods

PRODUCT	UNIT	GRAMS LACTOSE
Acidophilus milk	1 cup	11–13
Buttermilk	1 cup	9–11
Chocolate milk	1 cup	10–12
Dried whole milk	1 cup	48
Eggnog	1 cup	14
Evaporated milk	1 cup	20
Goat's milk	1 cup	9.4
Human milk	1 cup	13.8
Low-fat milk	1 cup	9–13
Low-sodium milk	1 cup	9
Non-fat dry milk	1.5 cups	46
Skim milk	1 cup	12–14
Sweetened condensed milk	1 cup	35
Whole milk	1 cup	11–13
Butter	1 teaspoon	0.06
Butter	2 pats	0.1
Half-and-half	1 tablespoon	0.6
Heavy whipped cream	1/2 cup	3.1
Light cream	1 tablespoon	0.6
Margarine	1 teaspoon	0.9
Sour cream	1/2 cup	3.2
Whipped cream	1 tablespoon	0.4
Yogurt	1 cup	10–15
American cheese, processed	1 ounce	0.5
Blue cheese	1 ounce	0.7
Camembert	1 ounce	0.1
Cheddar	1 ounce	0.5
Colby	1 ounce	0.7
Cream cheese	1 ounce	0.8

PRODUCT	UNIT	GRAMS LACTOSE
Edam	1 ounce	1.4
Gouda	1 ounce	0.6
Mozzarella (low moisture)	1 ounce	0.3
Muenster	1 ounce	2.8
Parmesan	1 ounce	0.8
Neufchatel	1 ounce	0.4–1.5
Pimento processed	1 ounce	0.5–1.7
Provolone	1 ounce	2.1
Ricotta	1 ounce	2.5–3.0
Swiss	1 ounce	0.5
Swiss processed	1 ounce	0.5
Velveeta	1 ounce	9.3
Cottage cheese	1 cup	5–6
Dry curd cottage cheese	1 cup	2
Low-fat cottage cheese	1 cup	7
Fudge bar	1	4.9
Ice-cream sandwich	1	2.4
Ice milk (vanilla)	1 cup	10
Ice cream (vanilla)	1 cup	9
Orange cream bar	1	3.1
Orange sherbet	1 cup	4
Soft ice cream (vanilla)	1 cup	9

best to eliminate all allergens as much as possible, and this means eliminating all milk and dairy products in your child's diet for now.

Besides looking for and avoiding milk products, there are several milk proteins, which may be added ingredients in processed foods, that will cause an allergic reaction. The most offensive ones seem to be *casein, lactalbumin,* and *lactoglobulin.*

After reading many ingredient labels, you will notice that a majority of nondairy food items do contain milk proteins. Casein seems to be the most popular choice. This means that most, if not all, nondairy products will not be appropriate for your allergic child.

Enzyme additives, which purport to make milk more digestible do not alter, reduce, or eliminate milk proteins in any way. These added enzymes only hydrolyze lactose. Therefore, enzyme-treated milk products will not be appropriate for your child. There are some infant formulas that are completely prehydrolyzed, meaning that all the carbohydrates and all the proteins have been broken down for complete digestion. These may be

---

Dairy Foods Containing Lactose and/or Milk Protein

2-percent milk	Half-and-half
1-percent milk	Ice cream
$1/2$-percent milk	Ice milk
Acidophilus milk	Low-fat milk
Butter	Malted milk
Buttermilk	Margarine
Cheese	Milk solids
Condensed milk	Powdered milk
Cultured milk	Pudding
Cream	Sherbet
Cream cheese	Skim milk
Custard	Sour cream
Dried whey	Whey
Dried milk	Whole milk
Evaporated milk	Yogurt
Goat's milk	

appropriate for your child in some circumstances. Otherwise, milk-free alternatives include soy milk, nut-based milks such as almond milk, and juice.

Are Nondairy Products Really Milk-Free?

There are a variety of so-called nondairy products in the marketplace that may or may not be appropriate for children with lactose intolerance or milk allergy. The government allows foods to be called nondairy as long as they are not made with dairy foods as we would normally recognize them. But that does not mean that these products are milk-free. For example, a typical "nondairy" creamer may contain whey (which includes both lactose and milk protein) or sodium caseinate (a milk protein). The FDA permits this product to be called nondairy creamer, however, because it does not have any cream in it.

Some of these nondairy foods may be perfectly all right, especially for lactose-intolerant children. Many of these products rely on dairy proteins such as casein as a main or substantive

---

Additives to Avoid as Sources of Lactose and Milk Protein

Casein—a milk protein

Lactalbumin—a milk protein

Lactoglobulin—a milk protein

Sodium caseinate—a milk protein

Calcium caseinate—a milk protein

Whey—contains both lactose and milk protein

Lactose—milk sugar

ingredient, but do not contain lactose. An example of this may be a nondairy whipped topping. Often these products contain casein (a milk protein) but no lactose and are comfortably digested by lactose-intolerant children.

The child with milk-protein allergy may not be able to tolerate many nondairy products because casein and whey, which are popular ingredients in these products, do contain milk proteins. Similarly, milk proteins have been known to show up in hot dogs, canned tuna fish, and a countless number of prepared foods such as packaged gravies, frozen dinners, and fat-free foods. Therefore, label reading can never be discarded by the conscien-

---

Nondairy Foods Containing Lactose and/or Milk Protein

Au gratin potatoes	Creamy casseroles
Biscuits, rolls, breads, buns	Creamy salad dressing
Bisques	Donuts
Breaded meats and seafood	Eggnog
Breaded vegetables	Instant potatoes
Breading mixes	Macaroni and cheese
Butter sauce	Mousse
Cake, pie, pudding, cookie mixes	Omelettes
Cheese sauce	Pancakes, crepes, waffles
Chowder	Pasta with cream sauce
Cookies, cakes	Processed meats (bologna, hot dog) unless specified kosher
Crackers	
Cream pie	Scalloped potatoes
Cream sauce	Strudel, pastry
Creamed eggs	Twice-baked potatoes
Creamed soups	

tious shopper. To help with this task, see Table 2.2 for a list of additives that may sound like lactose or milk protein, but are not.

Is Yogurt Safe for My Child?

Yogurt is a food phenomenon enjoying renewed interest these days. It's certainly an old food, having been around for at least four thousand years as a staple of the Middle Eastern diet. It's been both respected as a health food and maligned as quack medicine. But is it an appropriate food for children with lactose intolerance or milk allergy? Let's take a closer look.

Yogurt begins as milk. It may be made from cow's milk, goat's milk, or even from camel or sheep milk. It contains about the same amount of lactose as cow's milk, approximately ten to fifteen grams per eight-ounce serving. However, some studies have shown that yogurt may be easier for the lactose-intolerant person to digest than milk because it is partially hydrolyzed—that is, some of the lactose is already broken down. During the culturing process live and active bacteria are added. These bacteria actually hydrolyze some of the lactose, and if treated properly, may remain to continue their work when the yogurt is eaten.

Yogurt is produced by adding *Lactobacillus bulgaricus* and *Streptococcus thermophilus* to the milk, which is then warmed for a few hours. Sometimes the bacteria *Lactobacillus acidophilus* is used to culture products as well. As the bacteria multiply, the milk curdles and some of its lactose is converted to lactic acid. It is the lactic acid that gives yogurt its tangy taste. The bacteria then produce the enzyme *beta-galactosidase*, which presumably helps break down lactose further in the gut of the person eating the yogurt.

But here's the rub: Even though all yogurt begins with these live and active cultures, not all yogurts retain the healthful bacteria. Some products are heat-treated after fermentation, thus killing most of the cultures and eliminating their enzyme activity.

Table 2.2   Additives That Sound Like Lactose or Milk Protein, but Are Not Hidden Milk

Chemical Name	Is It Milk?	
Alginate	No	(seaweed)
Alpha tocopherol	No	(vitamin E)
Artificial coloring	No	(synthetic chemicals)
Artificial flavoring	No	
Ascorbic acid	No	(vitamin C)
Aspartame	No	(amino acid)
Beta carotene	No	(vitamin A)
Brominated vegetable oil	No	(designated unsafe)
BHA	No	(designated unsafe)
BHT	No	(designated unsafe)
Caffeine	No	
Calcium propionate	No	(calcium)
Calcium stearoyl lactylate	No	(calcium)
Carrageenan	No	(seaweed)
Citric acid	No	(citrus fruit)
Corn syrup	No	(cornstarch)
Dextrose	No	(sugar)
EDTA	No	(acid)
Ferrous gluconate	No	(salt compound)
Fumaric acid	No	(acid)
Gelatin	No	(animal protein)
Glucose	No	(sugar)
Glycerin	No	(fat derivative)
Gums	No	(plant derivative)
Heptyl paraben	No	(acid derivative)
Hydrogenated vegetable oil	No	(treated oil)
Hydrolyzed vegetable protein	No	(soy)
Invert sugar	No	(dextrose/sucrose)

CHEMICAL NAME	IS IT MILK?	
Lactic acid	No	(acid)
Lecithin	No	(choline)
Mannitol	No	(sugar alcohol)
Mono-diglycerides	No	(fatty acid)
MSG	No	(salt/acid)
Phosphoric acid	No	(phosphates)
Polysorbate 60	No	(sorbitol)
Propyl gallate	No	(designated unsafe)
Saccharin	No	
Sodium benzoate	No	(sodium derivative)
Sodium chloride	No	(salt)
Sodium nitrate	No	(salt derivative)
Sodium nitrite	No	(salt derivative)
Sodium propionate	No	(calcium)
Sodium stearoyl lactylate	No	(calcium)
Sorbic acid	No	(plant acid)
Sorbitol	No	(fruit sugar)
Starch	No	(vegetable derivative)
Sucrose	No	(sugar)
Sulfur dioxide	No	(sodium derivative)

Others may lose live and active cultures through the freezing process. Furthermore, not all yogurts are processed with the same levels of bacteria to start with. Currently, the government requires fermentation with at least two types of bacteria, but does not specify the level of bacteria manufacturers must use. In order to maintain live and active cultures in the product, fully ten million organisms per gram are required at the time of consumption.

In addition, many yogurt products on the market contain added milk, whey, or nonfat milk solids, raising the lactose content even further. This is especially true of frozen and nonfat yogurt. One exception to this is frozen yogurt manufactured by Colombo products, which distributes soft-serve frozen yogurt to yogurt vendors all across the country. The company maintains that their yogurt and frozen yogurt products do contain the optimum live and active culture levels.

To help lactose-intolerant and other consumers choose the most reliable yogurt products available, the National Yogurt Association (NYA), a nonprofit organization that represents manufacturers and marketers of live and active culture yogurt products, has recently established a seal of identification that can be seen on many products in the marketplace. The NYA "live and active cultures" seal guarantees that the yogurt product contains at least ten million organisms per gram at the time of consumption, the optimum number of bacteria needed for some lactose hydrolysis.

The lactose-intolerant child may be able to eat small quantities of yogurt without digestive upset. Depending upon his or her tolerance level, yogurt may be an important part of the child's diet due to its high calcium content. One cup of yogurt contains approximately 410 mg of calcium, over 100 mg more than in the same amount of milk. It may be helpful for the child to consume small quantities of yogurt throughout the day to garner the maximum amount of calcium while ingesting only small amounts of lactose to make hydrolysis easier. Unfortunately for the child with a milk-protein allergy, yogurt is not an acceptable food. However, it is possible to check for yogurt made from animals other than cows whose protein characteristics may be different and perhaps not as offensive an allergen.

Can My Child Have Chocolate?

Yes, your child can have some chocolate. There are many myths surrounding chocolate and dairy sensitivity. Many physicians and dietitians erroneously counsel their patients to avoid chocolate completely. But this may not be necessary. The confusion comes from the fact that often, outside of chocolate manufacturers, most people don't really know exactly what chocolate contains or how its ingredients affect the lactose-intolerant or milk-allergic child. Chocolate comes from the seed of the cacao tree. The seed, or bean, is husked and roasted, forming chocolate liqueur. Retain the fat, and the product is baking chocolate. Remove the fat (cocoa butter), and the product is cocoa powder. Add sugar, and the product becomes semisweet chocolate. No milk so far.

Up to this point, chocolate is acceptable for all dairy-sensitive children. Some semisweet chocolate may be labeled with a *U* followed by a *D*, a symbol indicating that the product is kosher (meeting the requirements of Jewish dietary laws) and contains a dairy component, signified by the letter *D*. The *D* in this case usually stands for the milk fat contained in the product or may indicate that the product has been manufactured on machinery also used for the manufacture of milk chocolate. Neither of these conditions should affect the dairy-sensitive child. Milk fat is the fat derived from milk. It contains neither milk protein nor lactose.

For our purposes, then, all pure forms of cocoa powder, baking chocolate, and most semisweet chocolate are acceptable. This makes baking and candy-making at home a real treat for kids who are dairy sensitive. Your child will be able to have all kinds of chocolate cakes, cookies, and candies made at home without added milk or milk by-products. Also, many semisweet chocolate treats may be available to your child at the candy store. Double check the premium brands, however, to ensure that they haven't added any cream to the dark chocolate blend. There are several chocolate syrups, morsels, and candies available at the market that are completely milk-protein- and lactose-free. Check for Hershey's cocoa powder, Hershey's Semi-Sweet Chocolate Chips, Hershey's Syrup, Baker's Baking Chocolate, Nestlé's Semi-Sweet Morsels, Queen Anne Dark Chocolate Cherries, Queen Anne Thin Mints, Mellow Mints Candy, Hershey's Special Dark Sweet Chocolate Bar, and Dove Dark Bar.

Kosher/Parve Foods Are All Milk-Free

Kosher (Jewish) dietary laws prohibit the mixing of meat and dairy in the same meal. Therefore all Kosher meats and processed meats are completely milk-free. Other foods that are neither milk nor meat are called *parve*. These foods are also milk-free. The Union of Orthodox Jewish Congregations of America marks all kosher food items with a *U* in a circle. If the symbol has a *D* following it, it means that there is a dairy product in the food or the food has been manufactured on equipment that is also used for dairy foods.

If there is a kosher bakery in your town, you are in for a treat. Kosher bakeries offer many cakes, cookies, breads, and rolls that are parve and, therefore, completely milk-free. As always, though, read labels carefully, as some unscrupulous companies may print the Kosher/Parve designation on food inappropriately.

How Much Food Should My Child Eat Every Day?

The United States Department of Agriculture in conjunction with the Department of Health and Human Services has developed new food guidelines based on years of government-sponsored nutritional research. The new food guide is called the food pyramid and replaces the four food groups guide, which was developed about fifty years ago. The old system relied on nutrition information now considered obsolete by current medical and nutritional authorities.

Many of you were raised on the four food groups and, as is often the case, will find it difficult to break old habits and change old attitudes, especially where food is concerned. After all, there is a strong psychological component attached to eating and also to feeding our children. We like to eat the foods we enjoy, the foods that make us feel good and give us satisfaction and comfort. We also enjoy reminiscing about the foods we ate when we were children and look forward to feeding those same foods to our children as a way of showing our love. Giving up or cutting back on the foods we love and learning to like new foods is a challenge for both children and adults. It is a challenge for parents who must help their children learn to like new foods, and it is a challenge for the children who need to have their diet altered substantially. But knowing what we know today about nutrition and health should make switching from the four food groups to the food pyramid much more palatable.

The old food guide emphasized the components of the system in the following order of importance: meats, dairy, breads and cereals, and fruits and vegetables. Americans raised on this system typically ate meat (or other high-protein foods such as eggs, poultry, or fish) with every meal, dairy (milk or cheese) at every meal, a serving or two of bread or cereal each day, and a serving or two of fruits or vegetables. But after years of watching Americans die increasingly from heart disease and strokes, government health agencies set about to study the cause of these deaths and concluded after decades of research trials, that three very important factors were contributing to the early deaths of Americans: genetics, smoking, and diets high in cholesterol and saturated fat.

The first factor, genetics, is something parents cannot change for their child, although sometimes even negative hereditary factors can be influenced by positive lifestyle changes. The other two factors, smoking and diet, are under the absolute control of parents who, by making appropriate choices for themselves and their child, can improve the quality of their lives and extend their life span as well. Over a period of twenty-five years, the government, in conjunction with university research centers across the country, has developed an appropriate food system and is now working to educate Americans about healthy choices they should be making, which include the cessation of smoking, the avoidance of a sedentary lifestyle, and the institution of a new diet that relies less on meats and dairy foods and more on grains, fruits, and vegetables. Parents who learn about the new dietary recommendations and feed their children and themselves accordingly will be setting the stage for longevity and good health.

Table 2.3 Daily Calories Required for Normal Adults and Children

CALORIES PER DAY	GROUPS
1600	sedentary women and older adults
1600	preschoolers
2200	children, teenage girls, active women, and sedentary men
2800	teenage boys, active men, and very active women

The food guide pyramid is built in the shape of a pyramid, with the foundation foods (those foods we should eat the most) on the bottom. These foods lay the groundwork for a strong diet. The other foods recommended are each placed above the foundation foods in order of diminishing quantity with the least desirable foods on top. The daily recommendations are as follows:

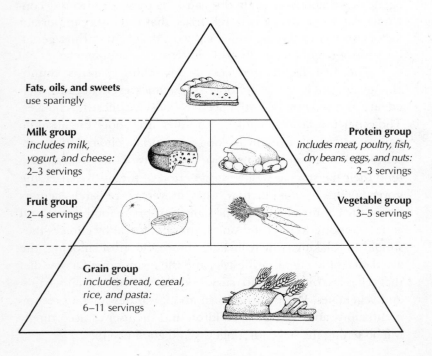

Fats, oils, and sweets
use sparingly

Milk group
includes milk,
yogurt, and cheese:
2–3 servings

Protein group
includes meat, poultry, fish,
dry beans, eggs, and nuts:
2–3 servings

Fruit group
2–4 servings

Vegetable group
3–5 servings

Grain group
includes bread, cereal,
rice, and pasta:
6–11 servings

Table 2.4 Sample Diets at Three Calorie Levels
Where Does Your Child Fit?

	1600 CALORIES PER DAY	2200 CALORIES PER DAY	2800 CALORIES PER DAY
Grain group	6 servings	9 servings	11 servings
Vegetable group	3 servings	4 servings	5 servings
Fruit group	2 servings	3 servings	4 servings
Milk group	2–3 servings	2–3 servings	2–3 servings
Protein group	5 ounces	6 ounces	7 ounces
Total fat	53 grams	73 grams	93 grams
Total sugar	6 teaspoons	12 teaspoons	18 teaspoons

HOW MUCH IS A SERVING?

Grain group: 1 slice of bread; 1 ounce ready-to-eat cereal; 1/2 cup cooked cereal, rice, or pasta

Vegetable group: 1 cup raw leafy vegetables, 1/2 cup cooked or chopped raw vegetables, 3/4 cup vegetable juice

Fruit group: 1 medium apple, banana, orange; 1/2 cup cooked, chopped, or canned fruit; 3/4 cup fruit juice

Milk group: 1 cup milk or yogurt, 1 1/2 ounces natural cheese, 2 ounces processed cheese

Protein group: 2–3 ounces cooked meat, poultry, fish; 1 ounce meat equals 1 egg, 1/2 cup cooked dry beans, or 2 tablespoons peanut butter

Average Americans then, including children, are being asked to flip-flop their typical food choices and select foods derived from grains at every meal rather than meats or dairy products. Now the bun is more important than the burger and the macaroni is more important than the cheese. That's a fact.

How much to eat? What constitutes a serving? Tables 2.3 and 2.4 are guides set forth by the United States Department of Agriculture.

3

Building a
Calcium Castle

Without a doubt, the most critical issue parents worry about when reducing or eliminating milk from their child's diet is the problem caused by taking away their child's main source of dietary calcium. Everyone knows that children need calcium to develop strong bones and teeth; without it, parents feel they will be putting their children at risk for poor growth. To be sure, there is reason for some concern.

Calcium is much like the water added to sand when making a sand castle. Too little water, and the structure will be weak and will certainly fall apart. But with adequate amounts of water, the structure will be dense and strong, and the sand castle will be sturdy and tall. Parents want to do the best they can to ensure that their children will grow sturdy and tall, and calcium plays an important part in the process. The truth is, calcium is vital to our health throughout our lives, and the more calcium children can consume and store, the greater their chances of retaining adequate amounts of calcium as they age. The good effects of calcium consumed by children last into their senior years when calcium depletion is at its highest level.

Understanding the role that calcium plays in growth, wellness, and disease requires a little comprehension of chemistry, biology, and physics. Most of us have no expertise whatsoever in any of these sciences, yet, in order to make decisions concerning our children's health and diet, we need to have at least some basic information about nutrition and the role that calcium plays in our children's bodies. First, parents can take comfort in the knowledge that no one food will ever completely ensure or destroy a child's total health. Nothing in nutrition is ever that sim-

ple. Present and future wellness depends in part on a complicated interplay of nutrients within the child's physiological systems. Under normal circumstances, calcium derived from milk
alone will not prevent your child from getting a disease, nor will
it cure your child of any disease. Still, calcium has emerged as an
impressive factor in many health situations and is most definitely
a mineral to be reckoned with.

Functions of Minerals

Minerals compose about 4 percent of each person's body weight.
Therefore an adult who weighs 150 pounds will carry about 6
pounds of minerals. Calcium and phosphorus are housed in the
skeletal structure of the body and account for about 75 percent
of the total mineral weight. Both of these minerals are considered major minerals for that reason. Other minerals held in
much smaller amounts in the body are considered trace minerals, although they are not necessarily less important by any
means. A deficiency of any mineral, whether trace or major,
could cause problems.

Minerals are maintained in the body by being absorbed
from the gut and excreted through various means, including the
kidneys, bile, and other intestinal and glandular secretions. It is
truly remarkable to realize that despite a constant flow of nutrients into and out of cells every minute of the day and night, a
homeostasis, or state of dynamic equilibrium, always exists in the
body, provided the supply of nutrients is ample.

Minerals are essential to the body. They form the greater
portion of the hard parts of the body including the bones, the
teeth, and the nails. They are components of respiratory elements, enzymes, and enzyme systems. Minerals regulate the permeability of cell membranes and capillaries as well as the
excitability of muscular and nervous tissue. Minerals are essential
constituents of gland secretions, and they play an important role

in water metabolism and the regulation of blood volume. In other words, minerals affect the actions of cells, nerves, muscles, glands, and enzymes. When the mineral content in the body is depleted, all of these actions and interactions can be negatively affected.

Mineral Composition of the Body*

MACRONUTRIENTS (MAJOR MINERALS)

Calcium	Potassium
Chlorine	Sodium
Magnesium	Sulfur
Phosphorus	

MICRONUTRIENTS (TRACE MINERALS)

Aluminum	Iron
Arsenic	Lead
Barium	Manganese
Boron	Molybdenum
Bromine	Nickel
Cadmium	Selenium
Chromium	Silicon
Cobalt	Strontium
Copper	Vanadium
Fluorine	Zinc
Iodine	

*Normal and Therapeutic Nutrition. 14th Edition. Corinne H. Robinson, M.S., R.D. New York: MacMillan Publishing Company Inc., 1972.

Functions of Calcium

Calcium's most prominent role in the body is to build strong bones and teeth. Fully 99 percent of the calcium in the body is held in our bones and teeth. Despite the way it may seem, bone is very active tissue, and the calcium in bones is always hard at work. In addition to framing the body, the bones recycle calcium reserves in the blood, thereby maintaining a proper blood calcium level at all times. This action is regulated by hormones and not food. Therefore, in this instance, the mineral levels in the blood are determined by the body's physiology and not by what your child had for breakfast. If the blood needs more calcium, it will be taken from stores in the bones to guarantee the homeostasis that is always maintained. For this reason blood levels of calcium will always test at a proper level unless something has gone wrong hormonally within the child's body.

On the other hand, calcium levels in the bones are highly dependent upon proper intake of dietary calcium. Here, the calcium your child ingests is vital to the density, hardness, and strength of his or her bones. While other factors do influence the amount of calcium stores in your child's bones, there is no question that food is a very important constituent in the process. Recent studies at Indiana University have confirmed that greater calcium intake among children will have a direct affect on the strength and density of their bones and the quantity of calcium stores for use later in life.

Teeth, like bones, consist of protein and mineral salts, mainly calcium and phosphorus. Teeth begin developing during the fourth fetal month and conclude calcification during childhood and adolescence. But, unlike bone, calcium lost from the teeth can never be replaced. So maintaining adequate calcium nourishment during childhood and adolescence is the first imperative for keeping teeth healthy throughout life. Growing children between the ages of six and ten need about 800 mg of calcium each day, the equivalent of the calcium in about three cups of milk. Teenagers require more, perhaps as much as 1,200 to 1,500 mg of calcium each day, the equivalent of about four to five cups of milk. When children and teenagers are on dairy-restricted diets, maintaining these calcium levels can be a challenge.

Outside of bones and teeth, the remaining 1 percent of calcium is in various body fluids. This calcium performs several functions. Calcium is vital for nerve transmissions and is directly related to muscle contractions in both striated muscles (voluntary) and smooth muscles (involuntary). Calcium activates an enzyme necessary for energy production. In the cells, calcium increases permeability, thereby assuring intracellular integrity. In the blood, calcium is a catalyst for the conversion of prothrombin to thrombin, a vital step in clotting. Calcium also plays a role in maintaining proper blood pressure.

None of this is shabby work. Minerals and water are excreted daily from the body, and they must be replaced daily through food intake. But which food? How much food? When to eat the food? How to prepare the food? Biology and chemistry aside, *these* are the most vital questions for everyday moms and dads.

How Much Calcium Does My Child Need?

Scientists who have studied the diets of ancient people have discovered that before dairying was introduced into the world, people consumed fruits, vegetables, and wild plants that were richer in many vitamins and minerals than today's foods. The researchers have even gone so far as to assert that before dairy products and grains became part of the human diet more than ten thousand years ago, hunter-gatherers consumed about 1,580 mg of calcium a day, an intake that easily exceeds current recommendations.

Table 3.1 Calcium Requirements for Infants and Children

AGE	AMOUNT CALCIUM PER DAY
up to 6 months	400 mg calcium per day
6 months to one year	600 mg calcium per day
1–10 years	800 mg calcium per day
Boys 11–18 years	1200 mg calcium per day
Girls 11–18 years*	1200 mg calcium per day

*Note: Some sources recommend 1500 mg per day for teenage girls.

Source: Food and Nutrition Board, National Academy of Sciences, National Research Council, 1989

Today, standards set by the federal government and other scientific sources can be used as guidelines for calcium intake levels. Sometimes experts differ with respect to exact numbers, and some sources list the requirements slightly differently, but basically, children require calcium in the amounts indicated in Table 3.1.

What Nondairy Foods Are High in Calcium?

Without a doubt, dairy foods are the most abundant sources of calcium in the western diet. However, milk and cheese aren't the only foods in which calcium is found. Calcium is found in several green and leafy vegetables, in tofu, and in some fish such as sardines and canned salmon. Calcium is also found in surprising places such as blackstrap molasses and mineral water. The following discussion introduces you to a variety of foods that will be important components of your child's dietary choices for nondairy calcium sources (see Table 3.2). A complete list of hundreds of foods and their calcium content can be found at the end of this chapter. Remember that one cup of whole milk contains about

288 mg of calcium. This will give you a frame of reference in evaluating the following nondairy food sources of calcium.

Casein-Based Milks There are several varieties of artificial calcium-fortified milks in the marketplace that use the milk protein casein as a base. The calcium content of these milks is often about the same as cow's milk. These products are not suitable for children with a milk-protein allergy, although they may be useful for children who are lactose intolerant. Some brands, such as Vitamite, come in both a liquid and powdered form.

Table 3.2 Nondairy Sources of Dietary Calcium: Calcium Levels Compared to Whole Milk

	Amount	MG Calcium
Whole milk	1 cup	288
Apricots, dried	1 cup	100
Arugula	3 ounces	300
Beans	1 cup	150
Blackstrap molasses	1 tablespoon	150
Bok choy	1 cup	250
Broccoli	1 stalk	150
Farina	1 cup	150
Kale	1 cup	150
Mineral water	1 liter	140–380
Okra	1 cup	150
Salmon (canned)	3 ounces	150
Sardines	3 ounces	375
Sesame seeds	3 tablespoons	300
Shrimp (canned)	3 ounces	100
Tofu	4 ounces	150
Turnip greens	1 cup	250

Soy Infant Formula   One cup contains 240 mg of calcium. This beverage is nutritionally complete for infants and may be suitable for older babies and young children when diluted. It may be used as a beverage or in cooking.

Soy Milk   There are a variety of soy-based milk beverages on the market. Some are fortified with calcium and are available in assorted flavors including cherry and chocolate. They are also available in aseptic packages, ideal for children to carry to school or day care.

Arugula   This lettuce is sometimes referred to as roquette or rocket lettuce. It has a peppery flavor and can be used in salads or sandwiches. Its calcium level is very high: 309 mg in a three-and-a-half-ounce serving.

Beans   Black beans, garbanzos, and navy beans all have about 150 mg of calcium in each cup. They can be prepared as soups, relishes, side dishes, or dips. When cooked beans are made into a puree, they can be spread on bread, crackers, or tortillas. A bean spread makes a wonderfully nutritious, low-fat alternative to mayonnaise or mustard on a sandwich.

Bok Choy   This is the Asian vegetable that can be eaten cold in a salad or tossed into any stir-fry meal. Bok choy makes a wonderful addition to the flavor of a clear broth. It contains about 250 mg of calcium in one cup, making it a very valuable vegetable calcium source.

Broccoli   Broccoli contains about 150 mg of calcium in each stalk. This vegetable may be pureed for infants and served raw or cooked to toddlers as a side dish or snack. It can be added to soups, salads, stews, and casseroles.

Kale   Kale is a member of the cabbage family. It may be eaten in salads, used to make soup, or cooked as a side dish. One cup contains about 150 mg of calcium.

Okra   One cup of cooked okra contains about 150 mg of calcium. It can be pureed, eaten as a side dish, or tossed into soups and stews. Okra has long been a calcium-rich staple of the American Southern diet, which incidentally contains many other nondairy sources of calcium. A Southern-style cookbook will offer many wonderful ideas for using several of the foods mentioned here.

Turnip Greens   These greens are low in oxalic acid and contain about 250 mg calcium in each cup. They can be cooked as a side dish, pureed, or blended with mashed potatoes. Greens may be used in soups or casseroles or eaten with other grilled vegetables in a sandwich.

Canned Salmon   Three ounces of canned salmon with the soft bones crushed into the fish will yield about 150 mg of calcium. Canned salmon can be made into croquettes or cooked as a loaf. It makes a wonderful salad and can be used as a spread for crackers or bread or as a sandwich filling.

Canned Shrimp   While not as rich in calcium as salmon or sardines, canned shrimp does contain about 100 mg calcium in three ounces. It can be tossed into salads, stews, or sauces. Blended with mayonnaise and lemon juice, canned shrimp makes an excellent spread for crackers or toast and can be used as a sandwich filling.

Sardines   Three ounces of canned sardines contain 375 mg of calcium. Sardines can be eaten whole or mashed and used as a puree or spread. They can be added to salads or casseroles.

Blackstrap Molasses   One tablespoon of blackstrap molasses has 150 mg of calcium. Molasses is one sugar source that has calcium and iron. It can be used in baking for frostings, cookies, or cakes. It can also be used to top oatmeal or pancakes. It can be substituted for honey in a variety of cooked dishes.

Dried Apricots   Dried apricots are a mineral-packed fruit treat. One cup of dried apricots contains 100 mg of calcium, 979 mg of potassium, 108 mg of phosphorus, and 62 mg of magnesium. They also contain large amounts of Vitamin B_6 and pantothenic acid, another of the B-complex vitamins. Dried apricots may be eaten as a snack, added to cakes and pies and muffins, or combined with several meat and poultry dishes. When cooked with sweet potatoes or white potatoes, dried apricots dress up and sweeten an otherwise plain dish.

Farina   The oatmeal of past generations, Farina is a grain product that is generally enriched with vitamins and minerals. It is made from bulgur wheat and is cooked and eaten like oatmeal. One cup of enriched Farina contains about 150 mg of calcium. Top with a tablespoon of blackstrap molasses, and your child will be consuming more calcium than in a cup of milk.

Mineral Water   Some mineral waters contain a fair amount of calcium. For example, Perrier contains 140 mg of calcium per liter and Mendocino contains 380 mg per liter. These waters may be mixed with fruit juice to make a cooler or mixed with fruit juice and frozen to make ice pops.

Sesame Seeds   These little seeds have a whopping 300 mg of calcium in just three tablespoons. They can be tossed into salads, stir-fries, and vegetable dishes or made into a terrific spread. There are a number of sesame seed candies available in the supermarket and in natural food stores. While they do contain some oxalate, these seeds should have a place in your child's diet.

Tofu   This is the "cheese" made from soybeans. Tofu is a white, creamy curd that can be eaten in a number of ways. Tofu can be diced and stir-fried or tossed into a salad. It can be pureed in a blender and mixed with fruit like yogurt or combined with spices to make a dip for vegetables or chips. Tofu can be eaten like meat in a sandwich. Four ounces of tofu contains 150 mg of calcium.

Calcium-Fortified Foods

Recent scientific evidence promotes the need for adequate calcium intake in childhood and throughout adulthood. Food
manufacturers have responded by inventing ways to fortify many
foods common to the western diet with calcium. These include
orange juice, fruit drinks, bread, soda pop, and even milk itself.
There really is no difference between consuming calcium-fortified food products and taking a calcium supplement, although
some foods, such as orange juice, do help calcium absorption
slightly. The body does not distinguish between synthetic minerals and naturally occurring minerals. Both types work equally
well in physiological processes. However, some people simply
prefer to take their calcium from fortified food products rather
than having a supplemental source, and parents may find this an
easier way of managing their child's calcium intake also.

Some of the calcium-fortified products in the marketplace
provide terrific alternatives for children with lactose intolerance
or milk allergy. The Lactaid Corporation produces a product
called Calci-milk, which is a lactose-reduced low-fat milk that has
been boosted with tribasic calcium phosphate, giving it 66 percent more calcium than unfortified milk. Calci-milk is expensive,
sometimes costing twice as much as regular milk, and may not always be tolerated by children with a significant lactose intolerance. It is also not suitable for children with a milk-protein
allergy. However, for those lactose-intolerant children who can
consume small amounts of milk without digestive upset, this
product can provide a calcium boost in their diet. To aid digestion, this milk can be consumed in small quantities throughout
the day, rather than in one large serving. Other dairy producers
are also experimenting with calcium-fortified lactose-reduced
milk. There may be several available in your area.

A calcium-fortified yogurt manufactured by Kemp's dairy
company is currently on the market. This new yogurt contains
about 800 mg calcium in one six-ounce container. That's a whole
day's supply of calcium for most children! It may be suitable for

lactose-intolerant children who can consume some yogurt; serve it in small quantities throughout the day for digestion without discomfort. Because this yogurt contains the full complement of milk protein, it is not suitable for milk-allergic children.

Calcium-fortified flours are now being manufactured by both Pillsbury and Gold Medal. If you use these flours to bake your own bread, each slice will contain about 50 mg of calcium. That compares to about 19 mg of calcium in a slice of regular white or rye bread. While not a significant calcium source, these flours are usually no more expensive than nonfortified flours and so are easily and cheaply substituted in all your baking recipes. There are also several calcium-fortified breads in the marketplace. These include Special Formula Hollywood Bread, which provides about 150 mg of calcium per slice, and Wonder Bread. The calcium content of these products is substantial. Two slices of calcium-fortified breads may contain the same amount of calcium as a cup of whole milk. There may be other brands available in your area as well.

One of the most sensible calcium-fortified foods available today is orange juice. Citrus Hill and Minute Maid are two brands easily available to consumers. Because calcium is absorbed well in the presence of ascorbic acid, or vitamin C, which is plentiful in orange juice, the two make a very nice combination. Typically, one glass of fortified orange juice will give your child the same amount of calcium as milk, about 300 mg per cup. Because orange juice is so palatable, practical, and versatile, it's no wonder that the calcium-fortified version has sold well. It makes a nice household staple and is readily accepted by the fussiest children and teenagers. Calcium-fortified orange juice can be served as a drink, can be frozen into juice pops, can be added to many recipes such as pancakes and banana cake, can be used to make sauces for chicken or fish, and can be made into sorbet. One cup of calcium-fortified orange juice combined with two slices of calcium-fortified toast for breakfast provides your child with about 75 percent of the calcium he or she needs for the entire day!

Other drinks that contain extra calcium include Tab made by the Coca-Cola company, and General Foods' Supri-Drink mix, which is a mineral enriched noncarbonated soft drink. Hawaiian Punch also comes in a calcium-fortified version as do Gerber Graduates, which are calcium-fortified juice packs designed especially for children. Gerber Graduates have as much calcium ounce for ounce as milk with no added sugar. There may be other calcium-fortified foods available in your local markets.

Is Calcium the Most Important Mineral of All?

Nutrition is an amazing interplay of vitamins, minerals, and other nutrients. The interrelationship between them is very delicate, yet very stable. Little particles of mineral interacting with minuscule particles of vitamins work just right to produce a healthy body. In order for calcium to work, it must be present with phosphorus, magnesium, vitamin D, and ascorbic acid (vitamin C). So it is important that your child receive his or her recommended daily allowance of those vitamins and minerals in addition to calcium. When planning your child's diet, you will want to include all the nutrients necessary for his or her growth and general well-being. Table 3.3 illustrates your child's basic nutritional needs.

Aiding Calcium Absorption

The single most important factor in the absorption of calcium is body need. Normally, adults who take in adequate dietary calcium will absorb approximately 30 percent of it, although some foods have an absorption rate of about 40 percent. Because their bodies require more calcium than others, pregnant women,

Table 3.3 Basic Daily Nutritional Requirement for Infants and Children

The following is not a complete list of all nutrients required by infants and children and is meant to be used only as a guide to your child's good nutrition.

	0–6 MONTHS TO 13 LB	6–12 MONTHS TO 20 LB	1–3 YEARS TO 29 LB	4–6 YEARS TO 44 LB	7–10 YEARS TO 62 LB	BOYS 11–14 YEARS TO 99 LB	BOYS 15–18 YEARS TO 145 LB	GIRLS 11–14 YEARS TO 101 LB	GIRLS 15–18 YEARS TO 120 LB
Calories	650	850	1300	1800	2000	2500	3000	2200	2200
Protein	13 g	14 g	16 g	24 g	28 g	45 g	59 g	46 g	44 g
Vitamin A	1400 IU	2000 IU	2000 IU	2500 IU	3300 IU	5000 IU	5000 IU	4000 IU	4000 IU
Vitamin D	400 IU	400 IU	400 IU	400 IU	400 IU	400 IU	400 IU	400 IU	400 IU
Vitamin E	4 IU	5 IU	7 IU	9 IU	10 IU	12 IU	15 IU	10 IU	11 IU
Vitamin C	30 mg	35 mg	40 mg	45 mg	45 mg	50 mg	60 mg	50 mg	60 mg
Thiamine	0.3 mg	0.4 mg	0.7 mg	0.9 mg	1.0 mg	1.3 mg	1.5 mg	1.1 mg	1.1 mg
Riboflavin	0.4 mg	0.6 mg	0.8 mg	1.1 mg	1.2 mg	1.5 mg	1.8 mg	1.3 mg	1.3 mg
Niacin	5 mg	6 mg	9 mg	12 mg	16 mg	18 mg	20 mg	16 mg	14 mg
Vitamin B_6	0.3 mg	0.6 mg	1.0 mg	1.1 mg	1.4 mg	1.7 mg	2.0 mg	1.4 mg	1.5 mg
Calcium	400 mg	600 mg	800 mg	800 mg	800 mg	1200 mg	1200 mg	1200 mg	1200 mg
Phosphorus	300 mg	500 mg	800 mg	800 mg	800 mg	1200 mg	1200 mg	1200 mg	1200 mg
Magnesium	40 mg	60 mg	80 mg	120 mg	170 mg	270 mg	400 mg	280 mg	300 mg
Iron	6 mg	10 mg	10 mg	10 mg	10 mg	12 mg	12 mg	15 mg	15 mg
Zinc	5 mg	5 mg	10 mg	10 mg	10 mg	15 mg	15 mg	12 mg	12 mg
Sodium	120 mg	200 mg	225 mg	300 mg	400 mg	500 mg	500 mg	500 mg	500 mg
Potassium	500 mg	700 mg	1000 mg	1400 mg	1600 mg	2000 mg	2000 mg	2000 mg	2000 mg

Source: Food and Nutrition Board, National Academy of Sciences, National Research Council, 1972 and 1989

nursing mothers, and growing children may absorb more than 40 percent of the calcium from their diet.

Interestingly, some studies have shown that as intake rises, absorption falls. That's because calcium absorption is controlled in the body by the hormone *calcitriol*. Low calcium intake raises the level of calcitriol, thereby improving calcium absorption. Conversely, high intake of calcium lowers calcitriol. Therefore, taking extra calcium above the requirement levels does not necessarily provide any value.

All of this is good news for children who need to restrict their intake of dairy foods. They will still absorb substantial amounts of calcium from the foods they ingest, even those foods with a relatively low calcium content.

Other factors influence calcium absorption as well. Vitamin D is important for calcium absorption. It is available synthetically, but it is also manufactured in the body through sunlight. Children playing outdoors during the morning or late afternoon hours are exposed to gentle levels of sunlight and benefit from the vitamin D garnered during the exposure. Calcium must also be soluble to be absorbed, and that means it must be well dissolved in liquid. Because acids help solubility, ingesting calcium with ascorbic acid (vitamin C) increases its absorption. Therefore children who eat calcium-rich nondairy foods would do well to consume them with foods rich in vitamin C such as orange juice or bananas. Citric acid, which is found in other fruits such as peaches and lemons, also increases calcium absorption. Certain sugars facilitate calcium absorption as well, including lactose (found in dairy foods), and cellobiose (found in cellulose fiber, a constituent of apples, beans, and whole grains, to name just a few).

Calcium absorption is also affected by stomach acidity levels. Reduced levels of hydrochloric acid can impede absorption. The mineral will be most readily absorbed when intestinal motility (movement) is at a nice, steady pace. Some sources conclude that absorption may be better during the evening hours when the gut is more likely to be at rest and motility is slowed.

Therefore, some experts recommend that children taking supplements do so with dinner or even later in the evening.

Children who receive the full complement of nutrients will fare much better than others when it comes to calcium absorption. So it is crucial to offer your child a variety of healthy foods each and every day and to see to it that factors that impede calcium absorption are eliminated from your child's lifestyle as much as possible.

Factors That Interfere with Calcium Absorption

Several factors will interfere with calcium absorption. These include stress, alcohol, tobacco, caffeine, excess fat in the diet, excess phosphate in the diet, and certain acids present in foods. Oxalic acid, found in dark green vegetables such as spinach, and phytic acid, found in the outer layers of grains, are substances which may interfere with calcium absorption. There is some controversy, though, because some sources claim the amount of these acids in foods is too minimal to matter and other sources claim they present a problem. Probably the best advice, then, is to continue to include these high calcium foods in your child's diet, but do not depend on them as your child's main calcium source.

The other factors listed above appear to indisputably thwart calcium absorption. While it may seem that some of these factors, including smoking and stress have no place in a child's life, the reality is somewhat different. While young children do not normally smoke, their parents or caregivers may, and secondhand smoke will impede calcium absorption. A child's life includes stress from the moment the child is born. Sometimes the stresses on the child are positive, such as excitement and enthusiasm, and other times the stresses are negative, such as fear and loss. According to the *Nutrition Desk Reference* by Robert Garrison, Jr., M. Sa, R. Ph., and Elizabeth Somer, M.A. R.D., "Calcium absorption may be reduced by physical and emotional stress, and may result in unexplained dumping of calcium into the intestinal tract. A net loss of as much as 900 mg may occur each day during times of worry and tension. Fecal excretion can be twice the dietary intake."

Other physical factors result in an excess release of calcium from the body. These are profuse sweating, excessive protein intake, and too much phosphorus in the diet. For many children, excess phosphorus in the diet comes from drinking too much soda pop or diet pop and eating processed foods. Studies have shown that diets high in phosphorus and low in calcium may contribute to significant bone loss. Excess protein intake is easily avoided through careful attention to a child's diet.

Calcium Throughout Life

The amount of calcium children ingest has a direct relationship to their calcium stores as adults. Children need to consume adequate amounts of calcium to strengthen their bones and teeth as they grow and also to store for future use by their adult bodies when calcium depletion from bones occurs normally during the aging process. Calcium deficiency has been shown to be a factor in many serious illnesses affecting adults including osteoporosis and hypertension. The primary target of calcium deficiency is bones, which become thinned and weaken significantly if body stores of calcium are inadequate. Recent evidence has shown that most men and women do not ingest enough calcium in their diets; at best, most Americans probably take in only half or two-thirds of the amount required. As a result, government agencies and health-care organizations have stepped up their efforts to alert people to the dangers of a calcium-deficient diet.

Helping Calcium Work for Your Child

The following tips will increase your child's calcium absorption:

1. Give your child an adequate amount of vitamins and minerals each day. Pay special attention to his or her intake of vitamins D, C, A, phosphorus, and magnesium.

2. Do not give your child antacids containing aluminum for tummy upsets as they will deplete too much hydrochloric acid in the stomach.

3. Too much fat in your child's diet will hinder calcium absorption.

4. Do not feed your child beverages with large amounts of caffeine. These include coffee and cola.

5. Some medications, including aspirin and corticosteroids, may interfere with calcium absorption. If your child must take these medications, be sure to compensate for the loss with added calcium.

6. Continue to feed your child spinach, rhubarb, and grains, but don't count on these foods as mainstay calcium sources.

7. Maintain normal motility of the child's digestive system. In general, this means that your child should eat sensibly and in a relaxed manner.

8. Understand that exercise is a must for all growing children and weight-bearing exercises, such as walking, running, dancing, and skipping rope, increase the density of your child's bones and muscles.

All About Calcium Supplements

Parents know best what their children eat and what their children don't eat. A diet of hot dogs and chips simply will not provide the nutrients children need. But should parents supplement their children's diet? There have always been two schools of thought with respect to vitamin and mineral supplements: those who approve, and those who disapprove. Many pediatricians encourage their patients to take supplements and readily prescribe supplements to children, especially those on dairy-restricted diets. Other pediatricians maintain that food should be the only source of nutrients for children who are basically well. But parents play a very important role in this scenario. They are, after all, the people who feed their children and are responsible for providing their children with adequate nutrition for good health.

My advice to parents is to always have confidence in your own feelings and impressions about supplementation based on your observations of your children's eating habits. If your children are poor eaters, how can they possibly be well nourished? Even good eaters often go through periods where eating nutritiously is about the last thing on their minds. During these times, giving supplements to children in recommended daily allowances will not harm their health and will protect them from nutritional losses that may be marginal, but will nevertheless affect them.

Studies show that parents who wait until their child's pediatrician discovers a vitamin deficiency may be facing a loss that is already well advanced. Sometimes months, even years, may pass without your child's body having the levels of a particular vitamin it needs before the deficiency shows up in a test. Some vitamin deficiencies, for example, a vitamin E deficiency, do not have any clear symptoms to identify them. But a deficiency in vitamin E could have a definite negative effect on the immune system. Many nutrients are stored for years in the body in surplus levels, but if not replenished, will eventually become deficient enough to cause health problems.

More recently, health professionals have become concerned less with outright vitamin deficiencies than with the effects of marginally adequate vitamin intakes. In other words, many children and adults are not dramatically deficient in vitamins or minerals, but rather are marginally deficient enough to interfere with normal body functions vital to maintaining health. These marginal deficiencies, often called "subclinical deficiencies," can be present in children who appear to be very healthy. In such children the processes leading to disease could already have been set in motion. Oftentimes, reversal of the disease process is impossible. Therefore, waiting to act until a clear, and therefore serious, vitamin deficiency is detected may not be the most prudent approach to your child's health.

Supplementation for children who are not consuming enough of the nutrients they need to grow and thrive will be a boon to their general health both now and later.

Let's face it. Parents only have so much control over their child's food intake. They certainly have complete control over their infant's food choices. And they have pretty strong control over their toddler's and preschooler's food choices. But they have less and less control over their child's food choices once that child enters school, and later becomes a teenager, capable of driving himself or herself to the local burger drive-through. Why not protect children with a vitamin and mineral supplement that will serve them well during the times of poor eating habits that they are bound to encounter? Two recent studies confirm that children who are well supplemented with vitamins and minerals do better physically and mentally. These children have denser, stronger bones, especially when given calcium supplements during early childhood. They also are better readers and therefore perform better in school.

What Type of Calcium Supplement Is Best for My Child?

If you decide that you want to supplement your child's diet with calcium, or other vitamins and minerals, you have several choices to make. The first question is which form to choose. Supplements are available in tablet, chewable, or liquid forms. The next question concerns the dosage. Remember that excess minerals are excreted through the urine and sweat. However, some vitamins, especially the fat soluble ones, which include vitamins A, D, E, and K, can be toxic at high levels. The best advice, then, about supplementation is to provide your child with no more than his or her recommended daily allowances given in a palatable form.

There are several types of calcium supplements available for children. Calcium itself is a mineral that takes many forms. It is a silvery yellow metal, the basic element of lime. When it is combined with phosphorus, it forms calcium phosphate. When it is combined with citric acid, it becomes calcium citrate. Calcium carbonate is a naturally occurring compound that is found in bones and shells. Calcium gluconate and calcium chloride are both used in the manufacture of medicine. Calcium hydroxide is a topical astringent. Calcium lactate and calcium caseinate are other types of calcium salts, and there are at least fifteen more.

When looking for a calcium supplement, it may be difficult to decide which one is right for your child because there are so many decisions to be made about cost, efficacy, absorbability, and practicality. Some forms of calcium are absorbed more readily, but are very expensive. Some forms of calcium are not as high on the list for efficacy, but are cheap.

As to which supplement is best based on its effectiveness, it is generally agreed among the experts that calcium carbonate and calcium citrate rank the highest. However, most of the calcium supplements in the marketplace today will do a fine job of delivering the minerals your child needs, with a few exceptions. Bone meal and dolomite are never recommended because they may contain lead and could therefore be toxic. In addition, studies have shown that some calcium supplements simply do not break down quickly enough to do any good. Presently, there are about four popular forms of calcium available for supplementation. They are calcium carbonate, calcium citrate, calcium gluconate, and calcium lactate. Some of these may not be right for your child.

Calcium Carbonate Derived from bones and shells, this is the form of calcium used in supplements made from oyster shells. It is also the main ingredient in Tums and some other over-the-counter tablets recommended as antacids. Generally, children will receive the highest amount of calcium per tablet with calcium carbonate, and it is easily absorbed and utilized by the body. Some people report mild constipation or excess gas as a result of taking calcium carbonate. But this preparation has long been recommended for pregnant women and children due to its simplicity, effectiveness, and safety.

Calcium Citrate This form of calcium is second after calcium carbonate for the highest amount of calcium per dose. Some studies show calcium citrate, which is the binding of calcium and citric acid, to be better absorbed than calcium carbonate.

Calcium Phosphate Calcium cannot be utilized in the body without phosphorus. Calcium phosphate blends these two minerals and is therefore a worthwhile supplement.

Calcium Lactate This form of calcium supplement has received some erroneous press lately. Some sources say that children with lactose intolerance should not have calcium lactate. This is untrue. Calcium lactate is the combination of calcium and a form of lactic acid, which is not lactose, but a by-product of lactose fermentation and other physical processes. Still, the problem with this supplement is that it has very little elemental calcium and must be taken in large amounts.

How Soluble Is My Child's Calcium Supplement?

A calcium supplement needs to be rated according to several factors. One is solubility. This refers to the supplement's ability to be dissolved quickly. In 1987 a yearlong study was conducted by Dr. Ralph F. Shangraw, chairman of the Department of Pharmaceutics at the University of Maryland. Thirty-five calcium carbonate supplements were tested, and eleven took so long to disintegrate that they were not sufficiently used by the body before being eliminated.

The United States Pharmacopoeia (USP) sets the standard of thirty minutes for total solubility. Of the supplements used in the study, only seventeen tablets dissolved within the first half hour. Some of them, however, disintegrated within ten minutes or less, providing optimum solubility. The top ten calcium supplements, based on their rate of solubility, are listed in Table 3.4.

Testing Calcium Supplements at Home

Obviously, your choice of supplement for your child will depend upon your child's age and ability to swallow tablets. Younger children will do very well with a product like Tums because they are easy to take chewables and come in a variety of flavors while delivering a highly efficient form of calcium. Older children and

Table 3.4   Solubility of Calcium Supplements

BRAND NAME	MANUFACTURER	% SOLUBLE/30 MINUTES
Tums	Norcliff-Thayer	100
Calcium Carbonate	Roxane Labs	100
Oyster Shell with Vitamin D	Nature Made	99
Supplical	Warner Lambert	98
Calcimax	Norcliff-Thayer	91
Os-Cal 500	Smithkline Beecham	91
Calcium 600 with Vitamin D	Giant Food	87
Calcium 600	Giant Food	87
Caltrate 600	Lederle Laboratories	69
Natural Calcium 600	Foods Plus	66

None of the following calcium supplements dissolved within thirty minutes:

Calcium 600-D	AARP Pharmacy
Calcium 600	Gray Drug Fair
Natural Oyster Shell	Gray Drug Fair
Sea-Cal	Natural Sales
Calcium 600-D	Plus Products Pathmark

teenagers may prefer a tablet like the Nature Made Oyster Shell Calcium so that they *don't* have to chew up anything.

Remember to watch the Vitamin D content in supplements and do not double dose this vitamin, because it can build up over time and become toxic. If your child is taking a multi-vitamin tablet with vitamin D, be sure the calcium supplement does not also contain vitamin D.

To test your choice for solubility, place the calcium supplement tablet into a clear glass, and cover with one-fourth cup of hot water. Shake or stir for a minute or two. Repeat this every fifteen minutes over the course of an hour. If the tablet dissolves in less than two to four hours, it is probably fine. Or, drop your tablet into a glass of vinegar. If it hasn't dissolved after thirty minutes, it isn't dissolving quickly enough to be used well by the body.

Medications That Deplete the Body of Calcium

Several types of medication will cause the body to release calcium or will interfere with the absorption of this mineral. If your child is on medication, you will need to supplement accordingly. Check with your child's pediatrician or pharmacist for more information. The following is only a partial list to consider:

Prednisone   Glucocorticoid steroids used for the control of severe allergies, lupus, scleroderma, some forms of Crohn's disease or ulcerative colitis, and rheumatoid arthritis.

Phenobarbital   An anticonvulsant drug sometimes used in the treatment of seizures or as a sleeping aid for infants or children.

Phenytoin   An anticonvulsant drug that may also go by the name diphenylhydantoin or the brand name Dilantin.

Primidone   An anticonvulsant drug.

Aluminum antacids   This type of antacid seems to increase the urinary excretion of calcium. One popular aluminum-based antacid is Amphojel.

Tetracycline A popular antibiotic that may temporarily cause some calcium depletion during treatment.

Warning: All of the above drugs are serious medications. Children who take them must be monitored by a pediatrician at all times. Parents must never attempt to alter their child's dosage of these medications.

What Other Ingredients Can Be Found in Calcium Supplements?

Pharmaceutical companies each have their own way of manufacturing mineral supplements. Some add vitamins. Some add fillers of different sorts and proportions. Some add colors and flavors. This is especially true for children's chewable tablets. There may be something in your child's supplement that he or she shouldn't have such as corn syrup or lactose or artificial colorings. Pharmaceutical companies are not legally required to list all ingredients, both active and inactive, on the label; however, many of them do so. Check the label of your child's calcium supplement, and ask the pharmacist for complete information, or call the pharmaceutical company directly if necessary.

Several vitamin supplements made especially for children also include some calcium. The following information should be helpful to you in choosing a supplement:

Bugs Bunny Complete Children's Chewable Vitamins + Minerals Manufactured by Miles Inc., these include 100 mg of calcium and 400 IU of vitamin D per tablet. This product is sugar-free.

Caltrate 600, calcium supplement Manufactured by Lederle Laboratories, contains no sugar, salt, or lactose and includes 250 IU of vitamin D.

Flintstones With Extra C Children's Chewable Vitamins and Flintstones Chewable Vitamins Plus Iron   Manufactured by Miles Laboratories, both do not contain any added calcium.

One-A-Day Maximum Formula Vitamins and Minerals   Manufactured by Miles Inc., includes 130 mg of calcium and 400 IU of vitamin D.

Os-Cal 500 Chewable Tablets   Calcium supplement manufactured by Smithkline Beecham, contains 500 mg elemental calcium per dose from calcium carbonate. It also comes in a vitamin D–fortified form called Os-Cal 500+D Tablets.

Poly-Vi-Sol with Minerals   This multivitamin/mineral supplement manufactured by Mead Johnson Nutritional Division, is a chewable supplement for children that provides iron, zinc, and copper, but no calcium.

Sesame Street Complete   This multivitamin/mineral supplement for children manufactured by Johnson & Johnson, provides 80 mg calcium and 200 IU vitamin D.

Unicap Jr. Chewable Tablets   Manufactured by the Upjohn Company, this product provides 100 percent of the adult RDA for almost all nutrients. It contains sugar and mannitol. The Unicap M mineral version of this product contains only 60 mg of calcium.

Other Minerals Are Important, Too

There is still much to be learned about the roles nutrients play for growing children, but we do know that a healthy child's diet includes a variety of nutrients derived from diverse food sources. Children need a full complement of protein, carbohydrate, fat, vitamins, and minerals of all kinds. The following guide should help you find other important minerals in foods your child will enjoy.

Boron   Found in fruits and vegetables, especially apples, pears, broccoli, and carrots, boron helps regulate the body's use of calcium, phosphorus, and magnesium.

Chlorine   Found in table salt and fish, chlorine helps maintain fluid and acid-base balance in the body.

Chromium   Found in meat, whole grains, broccoli, brewer's yeast, and fortified cereals, chromium plays an important role in the metabolism of fats and carbohydrates and in the action of some hormones, including insulin.

Copper   Found in shellfish, beans, nuts, seeds, organ meats, whole grains, and potatoes, copper helps in the formation of red blood cells and works to maintain bones, blood vessels, nerves, and the immune system.

Fluorine   Found in fluoridated water and foods grown or cooked in it as well as tea, fluorine helps form and protect bones and teeth.

Iodine   Found in iodized salt, seafood, seaweed, and dairy products, this mineral is necessary for the proper function of the thyroid gland, which regulates normal cell metabolism.

Iron   Found in red meat, leafy green vegetables, liver, peas, beans, nuts, dried fruit, and enriched food products, iron is essential to the formation of hemoglobin, which carries oxygen in the blood, and myoglobin, which carries oxygen to the muscles. Iron also is a constituent of several enzymes and proteins in the body.

Magnesium   Found in wheat bran, whole grains, leafy green vegetables, meat, milk, nuts, beans, bananas, and apricots, magnesium is vital to bone growth, basic metabolic functions, blood pressure, and the functioning of nerves and muscles, including the regulation of normal heart rhythm.

Manganese Found in whole grains, nuts, vegetables, fruits, and beans, this mineral is used for the production of energy and in building bone.

Molybdenum Found in whole grains, liver, beans, and leafy vegetables, this trace mineral is active in enzyme systems throughout the body.

Phosphorus Phosphorus is plentiful in many foods, including fish, meat, poultry, eggs, peas, beans, and nuts. It works with calcium to build bone and teeth.

Potassium Found in substantial quantities in oranges, orange juice, bananas, potatoes with skin, dried fruits, meat, poultry, and dairy products, potassium is vital for nerve impulses, muscle contraction, and the function of the heart and kidneys. It helps regulate water balance in cells and blood pressure.

Selenium Found in fish, shellfish, red meat, grains, eggs, chicken, garlic, and organ meats, selenium acts as an antioxidant in the blood, fighting harmful compounds, and functions as part of the immune system.

Sodium Although much of the American diet is too high in sodium, this mineral is found in table salt, smoked meats, and prepared foods, including baby foods. Sodium helps regulate blood pressure and water balance in the body.

Zinc Found in red meat, seafood, liver, eggs, brewer's yeast, beans, and wheat germ, zinc is important in the activity of enzymes, cell division, growth, healing of wounds, and other elements of the immune system.

Nutritional Wrap-Up

Table 3.5 lists a variety of foods and their calcium content. Use this information to help plan nutritious calcium-rich meals for your child.

Table 3.5   Calcium Content of Foods

FOOD	AMOUNT	MG CALCIUM
Meats/Poultry		
Beef	2 ounces	6
Bologna	2 slices	4
Chicken breast	1 ounce	9
Chili with beans	1 cup	80
Corned beef	3 ounces	7
Duck	3 ounces	24
Egg	1 whole	28
Egg white	1	4
Ham (boiled)	2 ounces	6
Hamburger	3 ounces	10
Hot dog	1	3
Lamb chop	1 thick chop	10
Liver (beef)	2 ounces	6
Peanut butter	1 tablespoon	9
Pork chop	1 thick chop	9
Pork roast	3 ounces	9
Salami	1 ounce	4
Veal cutlet	3 ounces	9
Veal roast	3 ounces	10

FOOD	AMOUNT	MG CALCIUM
Fish		
Bluefish	3 ounces	25
Clams (canned)	3 ounces	47
Cod	3 ounces	13
Crabmeat	1 cup	246
Fish sticks (breaded)	5 sticks	13
Flounder	3 ounces	15
Haddock (breaded)	3 ounces	34
Lobster	3/4 pound	80
Mackerel (canned)	3 ounces	364
Mussels	3 ounces	74
Ocean perch (breaded)	3 ounces	28
Oyster stew	1 cup	158
Oysters (raw)	1 cup	226
Salmon (canned w/bones)	3 ounces	167
Sardines (canned)	3 ounces	372
Scallops	5–6	41
Shrimp (canned)	3 ounces	98
Smoked kippered herring	1/2 fish	66
Swordfish	3 ounces	23
Trout	3 ounces	28
Tuna (packed in water)	3 ounces	17
Pasta/Rice		
Egg noodles	1 cup	16
Macaroni	1 cup	12
Spaghetti	1 cup	11
Spaghetti w/meat balls	1 cup	124

continues

FOOD	AMOUNT	MG CALCIUM
Fruit		
Apple	1	8
Applesauce	1 cup	10
Apricots	3	18
Apricots (dried)	1 cup	100
Apricots (canned)	1 cup	28
Avocado	1	22
Banana	1	26
Blackberries	1 cup	46
Blueberries	1 cup	21
Cantaloupe	1/2 melon	27
Cherries	1 cup	37
Dates (pitted)	1/2 cup	55
Figs (dried)	4	104
Fruit cocktail (canned)	1 cup	26
Grapefruit	1/2	19
Grapes	1 cup	15
Honeydew melon	1 wedge	26
Mangoes	1 whole	9
Orange	1 whole	54
Papaya	1 cup	36
Peach	1 whole	9
Peaches (canned)	1 cup	10
Pear	1 whole	13
Pears (canned)	1 cup	13
Pineapple	1 cup	24
Pineapple (canned)	1 cup	29
Plum	1 whole	7
Plums (canned)	1 cup	22
Prunes	4	14

Food	Amount	MG Calcium
Prunes (cooked)	1 cup	60
Raisins	1/2 ounce	9
Raspberries	1 cup	27
Rhubarb (cooked)*	1 cup	212
Strawberries	1 cup	31
Tangerine	1 whole	34
Watermelon	1 wedge	30

Soy

Tofu	1 cup	300
Soybeans	1 cup	138

Vegetables/Legumes

Alfalfa sprouts	1 cup	51
Artichokes	1/2 cup	51
Asparagus	4 spears	13
Beet greens/chard*	1 cup	144
Beets	1 cup	24
Black beans	1 cup	150
Black-eyed peas	1 cup	42
Bok choy	1 cup	250
Broccoli	2 stalks	316
Brussel sprouts	7	50
Cabbage (cooked)	1 cup	64
Cabbage (raw)	1 cup	34
Carrots (cooked)	1 cup	64
Carrots (raw)	1 whole	18
Cauliflower	1 cup	25

*Indicates oxalic acid present

continues

Food	Amount	mg Calcium
Celery	1 stalk	16
Chickpeas/garbanzo beans	1 cup	100
Collard greens*	1 cup	289
Corn	1 ear	2
Corn (canned)	1 cup	10
Cucumber	6 slices	8
Dandelion greens	1 cup	374
Endive	2 ounces	46
Green beans	1 cup	63
Green onion	1 onion	3
Kale*	1 cup	147
Kelp	50 gms	500
Kidney beans	1 cup	74
Kohlrabi	1/2 cup	35
Leeks	3–4 whole	52
Lentils	1/2 cup	19
Lettuce	1/2 head	40
Lima beans	1 cup	80
Miso	100 gms	140
Mushrooms (canned)	1/2 cup	7
Mustard greens*	1 cup	193
Navy beans	1 cup	100
Northern beans	1 cup	90
Okra	1 cup	184
Onion	1/2 cup	24
Parsley*	1 tablespoon	8
Parsnips	1/2 cup	35
Peas	1 cup	37

*Indicates oxalic acid present

Food	Amount	mg Calcium
Peas (canned)	1 cup	50
Peppers (hot)	1 tablespoon	40
Peppers (sweet)	1 pod	7
Pinto beans	1 cup	100
Potato salad	1/2 cup	21
Potatoes (white)	1 whole	8
Pumpkin	1 cup	57
Radishes	4 whole	12
Rutabagas	1/2 cup	59
Sauerkraut (canned)	1 cup	85
Spinach*	1 cup	167
Squash	1 cup	57
Sweet potatoes	1 whole	52
Swiss chard	1 cup	106
Tomatoes	1 whole	24
Turnip greens	1 cup	252
Watercress	1/2 cup	81
Wax beans	1 cup	63

Breads and Crackers

Food	Amount	mg Calcium
Bagel	1 whole	9
Biscuit	1 whole	19
Blueberry muffin	1 whole	54
Cloverleaf rolls	1 whole	18
Corn muffin	1 whole	1
Corn tortilla	1 whole	42
Cracked wheat	1 slice	22
English muffin	1 whole	96

*Indicates oxalic acid present

continues

FOOD	AMOUNT	MG CALCIUM
French bread	1 slice	16
Graham crackers	4	1
Hamburger/hot dog bun	1	30
Hard roll	1	24
Italian bread	1 slice	14
Melba toast	1 slice	6
Raisin bread	1 slice	18
Rye bread	1 slice	13
Saltines	4	1
White bread	1 slice	13
Whole wheat bread	1 slice	14

Cereals

All-Bran	1/3 cup	23
Barley	1 cup	32
Cheerios	1 cup	40
Corn Flakes	1 cup	4
Cream of Wheat	3/4 cup	40
Farina	1 cup	147
Froot Loops	1 cup	3
Granola	1/3 cup	18
Hominy grits	1 cup	2
Oatmeal	1 cup	22
Product 19	3/4 cup	3
Puffed corn	1 cup	0
Puffed oats	1 cup	44
Puffed rice	1 cup	3
Puffed wheat	1 cup	4
Raisin bran	3/4 cup	10
Shredded Wheat	1 biscuit	11

FOOD	AMOUNT	MG CALCIUM
Special K	1 cup	7
Total	1 cup	48
Wheat flakes	1 cup	12

Soups

Beef broth	1 cup	3
Beef noodle	1 cup	7
Chicken broth	1 cup	9
Chicken noodle	1 cup	17
Chicken rice	1 cup	17
Clam chowder	1 cup	34
Minestrone	1 cup	37
Onion soup mix	1 package	42
Split pea	1 cup	29
Tomato	1 cup	15
Vegetable beef	1 cup	12

Nuts

Almonds*	1/2 cup	166
Brazil nuts*	1/2 cup	260
Cashews*	1/2 cup	26
Peanut butter*	1 tablespoon	9
Peanuts*	1/2 cup	50
Pecans*	1/2 cup	40
Sesame seeds*	1 tablespoon	100
Sunflower seeds*	1/2 cup	125
Walnuts*	1/2 cup	trace

*Indicates oxalic acid present

continues

FOOD	AMOUNT	MG CALCIUM
Snacks		
Popcorn	1 cup	1
Potato chips	10 chips	8
Pretzel twists	1	4
Beverages		
Apple juice	1 cup	15
Apricot nectar	1 cup	23
Cranberry juice cocktail	1 cup	13
Grapefruit juice	1 cup	22
Grape juice	1 cup	28
Lemonade	1 cup	2
Limeade	1 cup	2
Orange juice	1 cup	25
Orange-apricot juice	1 cup	12
Orange-grapefruit juice	1 cup	20
Pineapple juice	1 cup	37
Prune juice	1 cup	36
Tangerine juice	1 cup	45
Tomato juice	1 cup	17
Vegetable juice cocktail	1 cup	26
Desserts		
Angel food cake	1 slice	32
Animal crackers	15 crackers	3
Apple pie	1 piece	11
Apple tapioca	1 cup	8
Brownies	1 square	8
Cherry pie	1 piece	19
Chocolate-chip cookie	2 cookies	8

FOOD	AMOUNT	MG CALCIUM
Chocolate-covered peanuts	1 ounce	33
Chocolate syrup	1 ounce	6
Donuts	1 whole	13
Fig bars	2 bars	22
Fruitcake	1 slice	11
Gelatin dessert	1 cup	34
Gingerbread	1 piece	57
Lemon meringue pie	1 piece	17
Marshmallows	1 ounce	5
Milk chocolate	1 ounce	65
Mince pie	1 piece	38
Mints	1 ounce	4
Pecan pie	1 piece	55
Pound cake	1 slice	6
Pumpkin pie	1 piece	66
Sandwich cookie	1 cookie	1
Sponge cake	1 slice	20
Yellow cake	1 slice	39

Fast Food

Bean burrito	1 whole	100
Beef burrito	1 whole	75
Chicken sandwich	1 whole	123
Chicken sticks	6 pieces	20
Fish sandwich	1 whole	60
French fries	small	19
French fries	large	26
Fruit pies	1 whole	10
Hamburger	1	50
Hash browns	small	25

continues

Food	Amount	mg Calcium
Onion rings	small	20
Quarter pound burger	1 whole	50
Roast beef sandwich	1 whole	40
Salad	1 small	22
Scrambled eggs/sausage	1 meal	75
Baking Needs		
All-purpose flour	1 cup	18
Baking chocolate	1 ounce	22
Brown sugar	1 cup	187
Buckwheat flour	1 cup	78
Cornmeal	1 cup	24
Molasses	1 tablespoon	33
Molasses (blackstrap)	1 tablespoon	137
Self-rising flour	1 cup	331
Semi-sweet chocolate	1 cup	51
Whole wheat flour	1 cup	49

4 Feeding Your Child at Home

One thing you can be sure of when it comes to feeding your child: Ask your friends and family for advice and suddenly everyone is an expert. Great-grandma will tell you that nursing is the only way to feed a baby. She might also tell you that holding your baby between feedings will spoil him. Your grandmother might tell you that your two-year-old is exactly the same kind of fussy eater you were. She might also tell you that you were completely toilet trained at sixteen months old and that twilight sleep is the best way to give birth. Your mother might tell you that you cannot raise a healthy child without milk. She might also tell you that the bacon and eggs and whole milk she fed you every morning at breakfast was the healthiest way to begin each and every day.

The point is, young parents need advice from others who have been there, and for the most part the advice is well-meaning and may be perfectly useful. But, as parents, you will be making the final decisions about your child's food, schooling, and play activities, as well as choosing methods of discipline and creating a general household atmosphere that is right for you. You may draw upon the help and advice of your family and friends as well as that of experts such as doctors, teachers, and authors, but you are ultimately responsible for defining your child's lifestyle. Learning as much as you can about aspects of child rearing will help you feel comfortable enough and confident enough to make appropriate choices for the well-being of your child. Feel free to talk things over with grandma, just don't make her your only source of information.

Children are obviously all very different from one another: They are individuals with their own emotional and physical responses and they grow up in households as diverse as the stars in the sky. There cannot possibly be one completely right way to raise a child. What is appropriate in one household may be inappropriate in another household. For that matter, what is appropriate in one five-minute interval in one household may be inappropriate in the next five-minute interval in that same household! Without a doubt, the most unwavering requirement children demand of their parents is flexibility. This is especially true when it comes to feeding. And it is doubly true when it comes to feeding the dairy-sensitive child, whose physical needs may change from day to day, or even hour to hour.

All families have their feeding rituals. Some parents demand that children take a bite of every food put on their plate. Some parents demand that children finish every morsel of food put on their plate. Some parents let children decide what the menu should be. Some parents make four different dishes for the same meal. Some parents turn meals into a holiday. Others turn them into a war.

This chapter will introduce you to various choices available for feeding your children at different stages of their lives and will offer you the best advice possible today, based on a combination of contemporary medical science and ancient wisdom. Please use this information to make decisions confidently, bearing in mind that without milk and other dairy foods in your child's diet, he or she will most assuredly be eating differently than many other children you encounter. Your child may be eating differently than you, or your mother, or your neighbor's child. But take heart in knowing that armed with good information and new options in the marketplace, you can raise your child on a dairy-free diet and your child will still grow up, be healthy and thrive.

Feeding in Infancy

In the west today, an infant eats either breast milk or commercially prepared formula. All experts agree that breast milk, laden with healthy constituents passed on from mother to child, is by far the best food for infants. Nature has provided breast milk with vitamins and minerals, water and fat, protein and folic acid—all essential nutrients for an infant's explosive growth. Breast milk also contains valuable antibodies that are passed from mother to baby and protect the child from a variety of diseases. Breast-feeding offers an opportunity for close bonding between mother and child and provides the easiest method of food preparation ever devised for feeding infants—no buying, no mixing, no storing, no warming. Physicians agree that all infants should be offered breast milk, regardless of whether there is a history of milk-protein allergy or lactose intolerance in the family. The prevailing thought is that infants fed at the breast for even a short time will reap important benefits.

It is true, however, that for a variety of reasons, many mothers choose not to breast-feed their babies. Their needs must be respected. It is also true that many babies cannot tolerate breast milk. Some infants develop an allergy to cow's milk protein and may not be able to digest breast milk, especially if the mother consumes dairy foods herself. Some infants are born with a lactase enzyme deficiency substantial enough that even the lactose in their mother's milk will be intolerable to them. So, in many instances—statistically in the majority of instances in this country—infants will not be fed at the breast, but rather, will be offered an alternative food source. In most cases, that source is commercially prepared infant formulas. Many options beyond breast milk are available to today's parents. This chapter will help you choose the appropriate food source for your baby.

Feeding the Milk-Protein-Allergic Infant

Cow's milk is the most common allergen in infants and small children. The offensive allergen is the protein in the milk. Cow's milk has about three times the ash (mineral residue) and protein normally found in human milk. This difference reflects the calf's size and rapid growth rate and proportionate demand for protein and minerals. Human milk protein differs in composition from cow's milk protein. Human milk protein is made up of about 40 percent casein, which is the protein predominant in the curd, and 60 percent lactalbumin, which is predominant in the whey. Cow's milk protein is made up of about 82 percent casein and 18 percent lactalbumin. The difference in protein composition alters digestibility. Casein is more difficult than lactalbumin for humans to digest, and this may account for the development of the allergy in a human infant who may have difficulty metabolizing the high level of casein in cow's milk.

Infants with allergic reactions to cow's milk protein may have diarrhea, vomiting, rash, coughing, rhinitis (runny nose), or eczema. If unchecked, an allergic reaction to cow's milk protein may cause asthma or anaphylactic shock, leading to death. Infants with cow's milk allergy must eliminate all sources of cow's milk protein in their diet until at least two or three years of age when a milk challenge may be done under the supervision of the child's pediatrician.

Cow's milk protein does travel through the mother's breast milk. Therefore, women who are breast-feeding their infants and ingest cow's milk protein will pass it on to their babies. A breast-feeding mother whose infant displays symptoms of cow's milk allergy should first eliminate milk and other dairy foods from her diet and watch for symptoms to abate in her child. If, after a couple of days of eliminating dairy proteins from the mother's diet, the infant's symptoms do not subside, the baby's pediatrician may perscribe an alternative milk-free infant formula. Most milk-protein-allergic infants can easily digest soy infant formulas, predigested infant formulas, or other alternatives discussed later in this chapter.

Feeding the Lactose-Intolerant Infant

As discussed earlier, most infants are born with enough lactase enzyme to easily digest the lactose in their mother's milk or even in cow's milk formula. But we also discussed the fact that the lactase enzyme is one of the last digestive enzymes to be produced before birth, and some infants are born early, perhaps several days or weeks before the enzyme has had time to establish itself in the small intestine. It is also possible for some infants to be born with a lactase enzyme deficiency, a condition known as *alactasia*. This is rare, but it does happen. Likewise, infants born with *galactosemia,* an inherited genetic defect, must not consume any lactose at all. Sometimes secondary causes may render your infant lactose intolerant. These include the development of an intestinal virus or another illness that causes digestive enzymes to be depleted or an episode of diarrhea, which can result from anything from teething to a milk-protein-allergic reaction.

Whether lactose intolerance is present at your child's birth or sets in as a result of a secondary cause, the symptoms are the same. Your baby will experience cramping, bloating, and diarrhea. Some infants also vomit frequently and will certainly have colicky symptoms.

Lactose intolerance is a reaction to the carbohydrate in all milk, whether it comes from a cow or from a woman. Therefore infants with lactose intolerance will react to lactose in either cow's milk formula or the lactose found in their mother's breast milk. Fortunately, there are several alternative feeding options available for lactose-intolerant infants.

Enzyme-Treated Breast Milk

Suitable for moderately lactose-intolerant infants
Not suitable for milk-protein-allergic infants

Mothers of lactose-intolerant infants who are breast-feeding might have good success using lactase enzyme supplements to treat their breast milk. The breast milk can be expressed and then treated with enzyme drops; this will hydrolyze the lactose from 70 percent to 90 percent. Some infants can handle lactose at this level. Another strategy is to cover the mother's nipple with liquid enzyme that the baby will ingest as he or she nurses. It is also possible to dispense the liquid enzyme to the baby through a medicine dropper just before nursing. Check with your child's pediatrician about the possibility of instituting this feeding approach and contact the manufacturer of the liquid lactase enzyme product for recommended amounts of enzyme to use with each feeding.

Infant formulas may imitate the composition of human milk very closely, but there are definite advantages to breast milk. It contains immunoglobulins and other substances that cannot be re-created in commercial infant formulas. These substances help protect babies from gastroenteritis and other infections. Another benefit of breast-feeding is the fact that breast-fed infants seem to develop fewer allergies to foods as they grow.

Studies have shown that some allergies develop because of premature exposure to foods and food substances and infants given breast milk as their dietary mainstay are often not introduced to potential allergens quite so quickly. Mothers who breast-feed usually have enough confidence in their baby's source of nutrition to hold back solid foods and other food products until the infant has reached at least six months of age. This practice seems to forestall the development of allergies.

For various reasons, some mothers choose not to feed their infants breast milk. They may be taking medication which, when passed through their breast milk, would harm their baby. Other women simply choose not to breast-feed because they are working outside of the home or because they are not comfortable doing it. While all experts agree that breast milk is best for a baby, they also agree that feeding your infant formula is still a healthy and viable alternative.

Lactose-Free Cow's Milk Infant Formulas

Suitable for lactose-intolerant infants
Not suitable for milk-protein-allergic infants

Your baby may do best if given a cow's milk formula that has had the lactose removed. Nutritionally close to breast milk, these formulas are based on cow's milk. They contain cow's milk protein, but the lactose has been prehydrolyzed, making them a useful alternative for lactose-intolerant infants.

Mead Johnson Nutritional Group recently introduced a lactose-free cow's milk–based formula called Lactofree. This product belongs in a new category of infant formula that is cow's milk based, yet lactose-free. There may be other such products available in your area. Lactofree and other products like it are not suitable for infants with cow's milk–protein allergy because the added enzyme does not alter milk protein.

Prehydrolyzed Cow's Milk Infant Formulas

Suitable for lactose-intolerant infants
Suitable for milk-protein-allergic infants

Prehydrolyzed infant formulas are those in which the lactose and the milk protein have both been predigested. These cow's milk–based formulas are suitable for infants with either lactose intolerance or milk-protein allergy. They are usually recommended for premature infants as well. Some popular choices are Pregestimil, Nutramigen, and Alimentum. Premature infants must be fed according to their pediatrician's advice with no deviation; parents of premature infants must never change their child's formula without medical advice. Some pediatricians prefer that normal term infants with lactose intolerance or milk-protein allergy be fed a prehydrolyzed infant formula. Likewise, this may be a highly suitable option for extremely sensitive infants or infants with a family history of allergies.

Soy Infant Formulas

Suitable for lactose-intolerant infants
Suitable for some milk-protein-allergic infants

There are a variety of soy-based infant formulas available today. Generally they are regarded as comparable to cow's milk formula with respect to nutrients and are usually well tolerated by lactose-intolerant babies. The protein and carbohydrate sources in soy infant formulas are vegetable-based and not derived from cow's milk at all. There is some evidence, however, that a percentage of infants allergic to cow's milk protein may also be allergic to the protein derived from soy. Estimates vary from as few as 10 percent to as many as 25 percent of milk-protein-allergic infants will react to soy protein just as they do to cow's milk protein. If this is the case for your baby, a prehydrolyzed infant formula will probably be recommended.

Soy infant formulas must not be confused with soy beverages. While these products may be useful for older children and adults, soy beverages are not viable alternatives for infants. They are nutritionally incomplete and inappropriate for infants. In February 1990, a severely malnourished five-month-old infant was admitted to Arkansas Children's Hospital in Little Rock with symptoms including heart failure, rickets, blood vessel inflammation, and possible neurological damage. According to the hospital, the baby girl had been fed nothing but soy beverage since she was three days old.

Please be sure when selecting a soy product for your baby that it is a complete infant formula preparation. Some brands available include Isomil, Soyalac, Gerber Soy, Mull-Soy, ProSobee, and Nursoy. Other brands may be available in your area. Check with your local hospital or pharmacist. Some soy infant formulas have added iron. ProSobee with Iron contains no sucrose. Nursoy with Iron has two formulations: one with corn syrup and one without corn syrup. The brand I-Soyalac is also corn-free.

Unconventional, Alternative Infant Formulas

There are several alternative infant formulas that are out of the mainstream but still may be suitable, and even advisable, for your infant. Some infant formulas are derived from bananas or are meat-based. There are even infant formulas based on chickpeas, a second cousin to the soybean. A chickpea-based infant formula is very similar in nutritional quality to a soybean-based infant formula and may be valuable for infants sensitive to cow's milk protein and soy protein.

Like soy beverages, goat's milk is never a suitable substitute for infant formula because it is nutritionally inadequate. Goat's milk lacks folates (folic acid), the building blocks of human growth. Also, goat's milk contains lactose as well as casein and lactalbumin.

Formula Preparation

Infant formulas are available in several forms: powder, liquid concentrate, and ready-to-feed. Any of these is suitable. Parents may select the form that fits their lifestyle most comfortably. However, proper preparation and refrigeration are essential. Opened cans of ready-to-feed and liquid concentrate infant formulas must be covered and refrigerated. Each preparation will indicate on the label how long opened formula can be safely kept for use. If you choose a powdered formula, the exact amount of water recommended on the label must be used. Overdiluted formulas will not provide the baby with adequate nutrition, although they may be recommended during times when the baby is ill and unable to manage full-strength formula. Underdiluting formulas will deliver inappropriate concentrations of nutrients for the baby's organs and digestive system and could put the baby in jeopardy of developing an irreversible disease.

Warming the formula does not affect its nutritional value, but many parents prefer to give their baby a formula warmed to body temperature. Some babies actually prefer their formula cold. This is a choice you and your infant will make together. Scientific evidence shows no nutritional advantage to either warmed or cooled formula. It is imperative, however, that warmed formula never be heated in a microwave oven; undetected hot spots in the bottle could seriously burn the baby. The best way to warm a bottle of formula is to place it in a pot of warm water for a few minutes or run it under hot water until the temperature is just right. Many parents will place the bottle in a pot of warm water while they prepare their baby for feeding. *Always test the bottle's temperature before giving it to your baby.*

How Much Formula Should My Child Drink?

In this instance, the answer to the question is based on a combination of solid medical evidence and ancient nurturing common sense. The answer is really "as much as your baby needs." No two babies drink the same amount of formula at each feeding. Pay close attention to your baby, and you will know when he or she is hungry. That's the time to nurse. If he finishes all of his formula, add an extra half ounce at the next feeding. But never force a baby to drink more than he or she wants. Ideally, many pediatricians recommend that an infant leave a small amount of formula in the bottle after each feeding. Then he is getting enough, but not too much. Your baby's pediatrician will help you learn the basics of feeding formula, but your baby will be the ultimate boss of his or her own nursing. After all, in nature, mothers nurse their babies until the babies stop sucking. There are no ounce measurements on breasts, and the amount of breast milk consumed isn't calculated. On their own, most babies take in exactly the correct amount of formula or breast milk they need to grow. Parents must respect their ability to do this so well.

Should My Baby Take Vitamin Supplements?

Now you are entering a sea of controversy. According to the American Academy of Pediatrics, "The normal breast-fed infant of the well-nourished mother has not been shown conclusively to need any specific vitamin and mineral supplement. Similarly, there is no evidence that supplementation is necessary for the full-term formula-fed infant and for the properly nourished normal child." If you notice, there are many qualifying adjectives in this statement such as "well-nourished mother" and "properly nourished normal child." What the statement means is that under the best of circumstances, all people in the United States should be able to derive complete nutrition from food. While this is true, we can all appreciate the extenuating circumstances that all people, including nursing mothers and infants, face, especially when it comes to nutrition. Not everyone eats well or metabolizes well.

This is why many pediatricians strongly favor vitamin supplementation for infants, especially breast-fed infants, who may not derive enough iron or vitamin C from breast milk or who may be nursed by poorly nourished mothers, who may not provide the infant with adequate amounts of nutrients. You, as the parent, may do well to simply comply with the pediatrician's advice about vitamin supplementation for your baby. This will help to establish a congenial relationship and demonstrates trust in the views of your child's medical caretaker. If, however, you have strong feelings contrary to the pediatrician's advice, you are entitled to enter into a calm and complete discussion about the pros and cons of vitamin supplementation with your baby's physician. The doctor should be able to substantiate his or her view on the subject to your satisfaction. If your infant is fed a well-manufactured commercial infant formula, he or she should be on a fine nutritional course, yet your child's pediatrician may still recommend a vitamin or mineral supplement for a variety of reasons. If this is the case you are entitled to know why the supplement is being recommended. After understanding the pediatrician's reasons, you may very happily agree that supplementation is indeed best for your baby. This is a challenge you will face again later, as your child matures and eases from formula feeding to table food.

The following information about nutrients a baby needs should help you determine whether or not additional vitamins or minerals are appropriate for your baby.

Iron   The amount of iron in breast milk is considered to be very low, actually 0.3 mg of iron per liter, compared to iron-fortified infant formulas, which contain 10 to 12 mg per liter. It is believed that infants absorb only half of the iron contained in breast milk, which amounts to about 0.15 mg of iron per liter, and only about 4 percent of that in formula, which amounts to about 0.3 mg per liter, and corresponds to complete absorption of the full amount of iron found in breast milk. According to the American Academy of Pediatrics, these amounts are adequate for the first four to six months. But your child's pediatrician may have his or her own view. While many parents complain that iron fortification gives their babies stomach cramps and diarrhea, scientific evidence so far has not borne out this fact. Still, many parents feel most comfortable feeding non-iron fortified infant formula to babies with frequent digestive distress.

Vitamin D   A deficiency of vitamin D can cause rickets, a disease that results in softening and bending of the bones. It is known that breast milk actually contains small amounts of vitamin D and so commercially prepared infant formulas add vitamin D to make up the difference. Still, rickets is extremely uncommon among breast-fed infants, perhaps accounted for by the fact that absorption is ideal when infants are breast-fed. Sunlight is also important for the formation of vitamin D, and babies taking in low amounts of vitamin D may benefit from a few minutes of sun exposure on their arms or face each day.

Fluoride   Supplementation of the mineral fluoride has been controversial for years. Yet the American Academy of Pediatrics recommends starting fluoride supplements shortly after birth in breast-fed infants, but also notes that nursing mothers who wait until the baby is six months old will do their children no harm. Currently there is no fluoride added to commercially available infant formulas. However, when formulas are reconstituted with fluoride-treated tap water, the baby will obviously be ingesting small amounts of fluoride.

When Should My Baby Start Eating Solid Foods?

The feeding habits of past generations have been quite varied with respect to solid food. Not too many generations ago, infants were breast-fed for one or two years before being given solid food. During the 1950s, it became popular to feed children cereal and fruit, which came from "cute little jars," and mothers were giving solid food to infants as young as two weeks old. Curiously, it was also during this time period that infant and childhood allergies began to skyrocket. Since then, scientific evidence has proven a definitive relationship between early feeding of solids and the formation of allergic responses in young children. Nutritionally, experts agree that there is almost nothing in solid foods that the infant needs if fed breast milk or commercially prepared infant formula for their first full year of life.

An interesting study of childhood allergies was conducted in Italy and reported in the *Annals of Allergy,* October 1993. The study, which was conducted on 158 newborn infants from allergy-prone families, found that careful diet helped prevent allergy formations in these infants. Mothers were told to breast-feed for at least six months and avoid eating a variety of allergenic foods such as eggs, tomato, fish, and nuts. Soy formula was used for any bottle feedings. Only 13 percent of the infants fed in this manner developed allergies, compared to 55 percent of infants in a control group not fed in this way.

This study seems to make the case for providing only breast milk or formula for at least six full months of your baby's life. It may be hard to resist the questioning and critisism of friends or family, but parents who avoid feeding their sensitive babies solid foods for at least six months will be enhancing their child's opportunity for continued excellent growth without promoting the formation of allergies.

The notion that feeding cereal to a baby helps him sleep has also been proved false. In fact, in some scientific tests the opposite has been proved: Early feeding, particularly of grains, which contain proteins and other constituents the infant's digestive system cannot yet break down, will encourage stomach upset and less sleep time. Furthermore, all babies are born with an involuntary action called the *extrusion reflex*. This reflex assures that solids forced into an infant's mouth will normally be spit right back out. So, your two-week-old baby is not really purposely eating the cereal you are feeding her, just sort of swallowing down the cereal by accident.

Young infants cannot yet communicate to their parents when they have had enough solid food because they cannot turn their heads away to let mom or dad know that they are not ready for the next spoonful or are simply not hungry any longer. When you think of it this way, doesn't shoveling cereal or fruit down your baby's mouth sound cruel? Your infant wants to nurse. It's something he or she can do expertly and the nutrition given through breast milk or formula is far superior to that of applesauce or oatmeal.

Current thought, based on a consensus of scientific evidence and common sense, is that infants less than four to six months old should not be given solid foods. The biggest concern among experts is that the solids will replace breast milk or formula in a baby's diet, thereby depriving the infant of its most valuable nutritional source. Some parents may want to wait even later until their babies can pick up bits of food on their own or have a couple of teeth in place. If your child is growing normally on an exclusively liquid diet, there is not much value to introducing solids too soon.

Special Needs of the Premature Infant

The premature infant is born with special needs in many areas, not the least of which is feeding. All decisions regarding your premature infant must be made with the help of your baby's pediatrician or other specialists. You may find a consultation with a dietitian helpful, if not now, as the baby grows. Being born too early means that some development of the body and bodily functions is going to take place without the natural aid of the mother. The baby is on his or her own, so to speak, to muster the energy that will enable him or her to thrive, to grow, and to develop normally. Prematurity has effects that go far beyond infancy, into later childhood perhaps, and parents are wise to seek professional guidance all along the way.

The premature infant is born with more poorly developed muscle tissues than its full-term counterpart, very little body fat, low stores of iron, and inadequately mineralized bones. The digestive system may not be quite finished yet and this limits the baby's ability to derive optimum nourishment from food. The premature baby's stomach is very small and can only hold a little food at a time, so feeding intervals must be frequent. Also, the digestive enzymes have not sufficiently developed for satisfactory digestion of carbohydrates, proteins, and fat absorption, rendering premature infants lactose intolerant and often allergic to milk protein.

Some premature infants have to be fed intravenously. Some may be breast-fed. Others require predigested infant formulas. Some are fed a combination of these options. Parents may not be given nutritional choices here, but rather, will have to wait to have some input until the infant has grown a bit. Without a doubt, breast milk can be a boon to your premature infant's nutrition by providing nutrients and valuable antibodies. Mothers of premature infants may need some help breast-feeding and should discuss this option fully with their child's pediatrician.

Will the premature infant become a lactose-intolerant or milk-allergic toddler? The answer to this question is not definitive. However, if cow's milk or other typically allergenic foods such as eggs or wheat are introduced into the diet too soon, the baby may develop antibodies that will cause an allergy to develop and possibly secondary lactose intolerance will ensue. If this happens, the gut may also be assaulted beyond repair, leaving it unable to absorb lactose, hydrolyze milk proteins, or utilize fat properly for a long period of time, if not permanently. Parents of premature infants must learn to wait until the time is exactly right before feeding solids or foods that are common allergens among young children.

Infants Should Not Be Fed an Adult Diet

A survey conducted on 1,500 parents whose infants drank the formula Similac revealed that parents wrongly presumed their infants had grown-up nutritional needs. The truth is that 40 percent to 50 percent of a baby's total calories in the first two years of life should come from fat. Most parents believe what they learn about their own diet applies to their infants as well, and therefore underestimate the vital role that fat plays in the explosive growth and development during a baby's first year. Fat provides long-lasting energy and is essential for normal brain development. It also facilitates the absorption of many vitamins. Parents do not realize that cholesterol in breast milk helps contribute to an infant's development and that infant formula provides the low fiber diet that a baby requires. Altering infant formula to try to make it low in fat is completely inappropriate.

Physicians at North Shore Hospital in Manhasset, New York, have studied several children who were admitted to the hospital's research center with severe growth problems. Fima Lifshitz, M.D., chief of the Pediatric Endocrinology and Nutrition Division, attributed the problem to babies fed on an overly strict diet. Some parents purposely watered down their baby's formula in order to try to cut back on the child's fat intake. Others refused to feed their young children snacks or meat. The lesson to be learned is that uninformed decision-making can be a dangerous habit. Please take the time to learn about your baby's nutritional needs and discuss the subject fully with your baby's pediatrician. Then you will be well equipped to make appropriate choices for your child. Please do not assume that the low-fat low-cholesterol diet prescribed for Dad who has high blood pressure is ever right for your baby. It simply is not appropriate.

The following dietary guidelines and Table 4.1 will help you understand your child's nutritional needs through the first year. But remember, this information is only a guide. Worry less about feeding your baby green beans at six months of age and concentrate more on establishing a relaxed and loving atmosphere in which to nurture your child.

Table 4.1   A Guide to Introducing Solid Foods

AGE	APPROPRIATE FOOD CHOICES
4–6 months	—Single-grain infant cereal including rice, barley, oatmeal —Fruit juice
6–8 months	—Infant cereal including multi-grains or wheat —Strained or mashed plain vegetables —Strained simple fruit such as applesauce or bananas —Fruit juice
8–10 months	—Infant cereals, all types —Plain regular oatmeal, Cream of Wheat, Cream of Rice, or Farina —Cooked, mashed table vegetables —Bits of cooked vegetables to pick up such as carrots or peas —Bits of soft peeled fruit such as banana, pear, peach —Fruit juice —Strained meats, egg yolk, tofu, beans —Bits of soft meats such as chicken, ground beef
10–12 months	—Infant cereal, cooked cereal, bread products, rice, pasta —Cooked vegetable pieces, raw vegetables as finger food —Mashed beans —Fresh peeled fruits, canned fruits packed in juice —Fruit juice —Egg yolk —Whole egg (at 12 months) —Peanut butter

Source: *Nutrition and Feeding of Infants and Toddlers* by Rosanne N. Howard and Harland S. Winter. Boston: Little, Brown and Company, 1984

Dietary Guidelines for Infants

The following guidelines were prepared by Guy H. Johnson, Ph.D., director of infant nutrition for the Gerber Products

Company, based on published statements from the Academy of Pediatrics and the American Dietetic Association.

1. **Build to a variety of foods.** Breast milk or commercially prepared infant formula should be the only nourishment an infant receives during the first few months of life. Between the ages of four to six months, begin introducing your baby to solid foods beginning with single grains and other single-ingredient foods as recommended by your baby's pediatrician.

2. **Listen to your baby's appetite to avoid overfeeding or underfeeding.** Babies should be fed when hungry, but not forced to finish formula in a bottle or the last spoonfuls of food in a dish. Babies who shake their heads no or spit the food out are probably full. Never force an infant to eat.

3. **Don't restrict fat and cholesterol too much.** Caloric requirements are higher during infancy than at any other time. And because infants have small stomachs, their food must pack a wallop when it comes to calories and other nutrients including fat and cholesterol. Sensible choices of solid foods along with breast milk or infant formula will provide adequate nutrition for your child.

4. **Don't overdo high-fiber foods.** Whole-grain foods and high-fiber cereals recommended for adults are not necessary for babies less than two years old. The fiber found naturally in many foods commonly given to babies, such as pureed fruits and vegetables or infant cereals, is appropriate.

5. **Sugar is okay, but in moderation.** Infants fed breast milk or infant formula will be taking in moderate amounts of sugar in several forms. The fruit juices and pureed fruits and vegetables that your baby wil be eating later all contain some amounts of sugar. The one form of sugar that is never permitted for infants is honey, which contains a particular type of botulism spore that may be deadly to infants because they are unable to defend against its harmful effects.

6. **Sodium is okay, but in moderation.** Sodium, a valuable mineral for all infants, children, and adults is naturally found in

almost all foods. Processed foods, with high levels of sodium, should be avoided, or only offered occasionally.

7. Babies need more iron, pound for pound, than adults. Normally, infants are born with a supply of iron that lasts for the first four to six months of life. After this time, iron must be supplied by foods in the diet. Especially good sources of iron for your baby are fortified infant formulas and cereals.

Feeding the Older Baby, One to Three Years

From their first to third year, most babies will be given whole milk in their diet to replace infant formula or breast milk. Your dairy-sensitive baby will most likely not be introduced to milk at this time. If your child is allergic to milk protein, it is commonly advised that milk and other dairy foods be withheld until your child is at least two to three years of age and then only given under a pediatrician's supervision. If your child is lactose intolerant, it is still inappropriate to offer dairy foods, unless you are certain that some may be taken without ill effect. For now, you will still be relying on commercially prepared infant formula or other substitute beverages available for the dairy-sensitive child. Later, when your child is more than three years old, it may be advisable to check for tolerance levels of lactose and threshold levels of milk-protein allergy. You will learn how to do this shortly.

Children between the ages of one and three should be eating a variety of foods including fruits, vegetables, juices, cereals, breads, pasta and rice, eggs, and meats. These will provide the child with the appropriate amount of protein, fat, fiber, and vitamins and minerals. Children of this age should also be feeding themselves, for the most part. Your child at even ten months old is probably capable of picking up bits of soft food and gumming them. Children encouraged to feed themselves gain a valuable sense of independence. Parents may need to do some fill-in

feeding, especially for younger babies, who have not yet mas-
tered the art of eating with a spoon. But even a one-year-old can
usually eat bits of almost anything—dried cereals, cut-up soft
fruit, eggs, vegetable pieces, cooked soft meats. Some young babies thrive on sucking and softening hard biscuit-type breads
such as zweiback, which melt in their mouths easily.

By three years old, your child will be so far advanced when
it comes to feeding him- or herself, that parental intervention of
any kind should no longer be necessary. Children this age can
eat with utensils, drink from cups and glasses, and eat at the
adult table. They can even set the table, clear the dishes, and
learn some manners. The essential role that parents do play is to
provide a home full of appropriate, healthy foods that are nour-
ishing and enjoyable to eat. Children who always have fruit in the
house will often eat fruit. Children who always have vegetables
served at mealtime will often eat vegetables. Children who always
have junque in the house will often eat junque. As parental control wanes and children help themselves to foods more often, it
is very important that the choices parents make available at
home be especially healthy ones. If there are no potato chips at
home today, no potato chips will be eaten by your three-year-old.

As your child moves out of infancy and into childhood, his
or her nutritional needs change greatly. In addition, the manner
in which parents approach feeding has a huge effect upon the
manner in which their children eat. There is an emotional component as well as a nutritional component to feeding one-to-
three year olds. To learn about both of these issues, we will
consult the experts, but still rely on the common-sense axiom
that all people are individuals, and none of what follows is a rule,
only a guideline.

Nutritional Needs of Children, One to Three Years

Children from twelve to thirty-six months of age, who weigh up
to about twenty-eight pounds, should be eating about 1,300

calories per day. They require a full complement of nutrients, including vitamins, minerals, protein, and fat. Children at twelve months of age will still be having about three to four feedings, or about twenty-four to thirty-two ounces of either breast milk or infant formula each day, providing nearly half of the calories they need. During the next twelve to twenty-four months, babies will be in a period of transition as they are first introduced to table food, weaned from breast or bottle, and learn to rely on table foods as their sole source of nutrition. Experts today do not recommend feeding children at this age on a strict "three meal a day" schedule. Snacks are just as important as meals and provide parents the opportunity to slip in some very nutritious foods in small quantities. Besides, children this age require several opportunities during the day to refuel in order to keep up with their high activity levels.

Based on the food pyramid guide, by three years old your child should be eating the following each day:

- Grain group, includes breads, cereals, rice, and pasta: about four to six servings
- Vegetable group, includes green and yellow vegetables, raw and cooked: about two to three servings
- Fruit group, includes fresh or cooked fruit or juice: about two servings
- Protein group, includes meat, poultry, fish, dry beans, eggs, and nuts: about two three-ounce servings
- Milk group: the equivalent of about two servings of dairy foods includes 400 IU of vitamin D, 800 mg of calcium, and 800 mg of phosphorus

To help select milk-free alternatives for these nutrients, the following suggests some good choices.

Alternative Beverages Instead of Milk

There are several alternatives to milk available as beverages for your child. Many of them have been fortified to provide some of

Nondairy Alternatives to Nutrients Provided by Milk and Other Dairy Foods

400 IU Vitamin D

Instead of two cups of fortified whole milk, choose the following:

A vitamin supplement

Several minutes of exposure to the sun each day

Cod-liver oil

Foods containing vitamin D including egg yolk, salmon, sardines, and liver

A vitamin-fortified soy beverage

800 mg Calcium

Instead of two to three cups of fortified whole milk, choose the following:

A mineral supplement

A combination of the following foods:

1 cup crabmeat (246 mg calcium)

3 ounces canned mackerel (364 mg calcium)

3 ounces canned salmon (167 mg calcium)

3 ounces canned sardines (372 mg calcium)

1 cup dried apricots (100 mg calcium)

4 dried figs (104 mg calcium)

1 cup tofu (300 mg calcium)

1 cup black beans (150 mg calcium)

1 cup chickpeas (150 mg calcium)

1 cup navy beans (100 mg calcium)

2 stalks broccoli (316 mg calcium)

1 cup bok choy (250 mg calcium)

$^3/_4$ cup Cream of Wheat (147 mg calcium)

1 cup Swiss chard (106 mg calcium)

$^1/_2$ cup almonds (166 mg calcium) (contains oxalates)

1 tablespoon sesame seeds (100 mg calcium) (contains oxalates)

1 tablespoon blackstrap molasses (137 mg calcium)

A mineral fortified juice or soy beverage

800 mg Phosphorus

Instead of two to three cups of fortified whole milk, choose the following:

A mineral supplement

A combination of the following foods:

1 cup dried apricots (108 mg phosphorus)

1 cup cooked lima beans (121 mg phosphorus)

1 small beef hamburger (194 mg phosphorus)

3 ounces lean beef (246 mg phosphorus)

3 ounces bluefish (287 mg phosphorus)

$^3/_4$ cup cashew nuts (373 mg phosphorus)

3 ounces chicken, white or dark meat (250 mg phosphorus)

1 whole egg (205 mg phosphorus)

3 ounces lamb (223 mg phosphorus)

3 ounces beef liver (476 mg phosphorus)

the same nutrients as milk. You will want to acquaint yourself with the variety of options available to you in your area by combing the supermarkets, whole-food stores, health-food stores, and checking with the manufacturers of commercially prepared infant formulas. Some of these manufacturers produce so-called intermediate drinks for children between the ages of one and three; these have been fortified to give them a variety of essential nutrients similar to milk. Some, but not all, of these beverages will be suitable choices for your two- or three-year-old child.

Intermediate Milks

Suitable for lactose-intolerant children
Not suitable for milk-protein-allergic children

There are several intermediate beverages in the marketplace, which are manufactured by the same companies that provide prepared infant formulas. Most of these beverages are milk-protein-based and also contain lactose. They are meant to provide adequate nutrients for toddlers, but with reduced calories and fat compared to formula, to take into account the toddler's slowed growth and the addition of a variety of solid foods to the diet. Many parents find it difficult to resist wanting to try these beverages, which may be advertised heavily in parenting magazines and other publications or on television shows geared to parenting. However, these products, for the most part, are not suitable for dairy-sensitive children. Mead Johnson's Next Step Toddler Formula, for example, is a milk-based beverage containing both milk protein and lactose. It is actually a poor source of minerals since it contains only 120 mg of calcium and 84 mg of phosphorus per serving. Carnation also manufactures a beverage called Follow Up Formula. This too contains milk protein and lactose.

There is one product available, however, that is lactose-free. It is manufactured by Ross Laboratories and is called PediaSure. This product contains the milk protein casein, but may be a very valuable milk alternative for toddlers who are lactose intolerant. It has been fortified to contain 230 mg of calcium, 120 IU vitamin D, and 190 mg phosphorus in each serving. The calcium content of PediaSure is very close to that of whole milk, and two or three cups of this beverage per day could be a valuable calcium source for the lactose-intolerant child. The

product is available in a variety of flavors including vanilla,
strawberry, chocolate, and banana cream.

Soy Beverages

Suitable for lactose-intolerant children
Suitable for milk-protein-allergic children
Not suitable for soy-protein-allergic children

The food shelves and refrigerated sections of supermarkets are
significantly stocked with soy beverages these days. While there
are some advantages to soy beverages for your child, there are
problems as well. Soy beverages are lactose-free and milk-
protein-free, but may cause an allergic response in the child sensitive to soy protein. These beverages are found in a variety of
flavors including vanilla, chocolate, carob, and strawberry, to
name a few. Some familiar manufacturers of soy beverages are
Edensoy and Vitasoy; both companies produce several types of
soy products. While these beverages may be tasty and will provide your child with a worthwhile nonmeat protein source, most
of the soy beverages are not terribly abundant in other nutrients
children need, including calcium. A typical serving of a soy beverage will provide a child with only about 80 mg of calcium.

One exception is a fortified product manufactured by
Edensoy called Edensoy Extra. This product, also available in several flavors, will provide your child with about 20 percent of his
or her calcium requirement per serving, about 25 percent of his
or her vitamin E requirement, and about 30 percent of his or her
vitamin A requirement. It is also fortified with a small amount of
beta carotene.

Parents who choose to give their children soy beverages
should not rely on these as substitutes for infant formulas nor as
mainstay calcium sources, unless they have been fortified. They
are, however, very useful as protein sources, especially for children who do not eat meat or eggs. They are also terrific dairy substitutes in recipes. Because soy beverages are often undetectable

in many dishes that call for milk, they may make a nice substitution in your family's favorite recipes.

Goat's Milk and Sheep's Milk

Not suitable for lactose-intolerant children
May be suitable for milk-protein-allergic children

As discussed earlier, goat's milk, and other animal milks, including sheep's milk, contain lactose and also contain the proteins casein and lactalbumin. Compared to cow's milk, one cup of goat's milk contains slightly more calcium, about equal amounts of lactose and milk protein, considerably less casein, and more lactalbumin. Goat's milk also contains more fat than cow's milk, although the globules are smaller, and therefore more digestible. According to the *University of California Berkeley Wellness Letter* of May 1988, about two-thirds of children allergic to cow's milk will also be allergic to goat's milk. If taken in an unpasteurized form, goat's milk may also contain more offending bacteria. It may be well tolerated by your child with a milk-protein allergy, but should not be introduced until after the child is three years old and can withstand a milk-protein allergy challenge.

Sheep's milk products are beginning to surface more and more in the marketplace. They have long been found in health food stores, but now are being stocked by several whole food chains as well as by major supermarkets. Sheep's milk contains lactose and the same proteins as cow's milk, but in slightly different proportions. Its calcium and phosphorus content is similar to that of cow's milk, and its fat content is much higher than either goat's milk or cow's milk, which makes the milk taste quite sweet. Some studies have shown that sheep's milk has properties that make it more digestible than cow's milk for children with allergies and intolerances. So sheep's milk may be useful to experiment with, but not before your child is ready to become involved in protein challenges. Small amounts of goat's milk or sheep's milk may be tried in lactose-intolerant children, but it should be immediately withdrawn if symptoms of digestive distress occur.

Feeding Your Child, Four to Ten Years

Typically, boys and girls between the ages of four and ten weigh somewhere between forty-four and sixty-six pounds and require between 1,800 and 2,400 calories per day. They need about 800 mg of calcium, 250 mg magnesium, and 800 mg phosphorus per day. They also require large amounts of vitamin A, between 2,500 and 3,300 IU.

Dairy-sensitive children of this age should be ready to be evaluated for their levels of lactose intolerance and their milk-protein-allergy thresholds. You may want more explicit advice from your child's pediatrician during this time, especially when dealing with the allergic child.

The diet of the four- to ten-year-old should be sufficiently varied and should contain significant amounts of nutrients to provide these children with growing power and the energy they need to cope with their energetic lifestyle. According to the new food guide provided by the United States Department of Agriculture, children in this age group should be eating the following each day:

- Grain group: nine servings per day
- Vegetable group: four servings per day
- Fruit group: three servings per day
- Protein group: six ounces per day
- Dairy group: the equivalent of two to three servings of milk per day
- Total fat: 73 grams
- Total added sugar: 12 teaspoons

Children between four and ten years old will be able to eat a variety of calcium-fortified nondairy foods. These include calcium-fortified orange juice, soy beverages, fruit drinks, breads, and dry cereals. Depending upon their tolerance levels, lactose-intolerant children may do very well with lactase enzyme–treated milk or with lactase enzyme chewable tablet supplementation.

These foods and enzyme products can be incorporated into their school lunches and included on other occasions when children will not be eating at home. Vitamin and mineral supplements, if used, can be taken in chewable or liquid form or swallowed whole. Even a five-year-old is capable of swallowing vitamin pills. Try teaching your child to swallow pills by using Cheerios—they're a perfect size and can be washed down very easily with a quick swig of juice or water.

Finding Your Child's Lactose Tolerance Level

As we learned earlier, lactose intolerance is a highly subjective condition. Some children can eat small amounts of milk or other dairy foods each day. Some children can have a small amount of milk two or three times a week without difficulty. Some children can't have any. It has been observed that, mysteriously, some children with lactose intolerance go through a sort of "remission" period and are better able to tolerate lactose during their middle childhood years. The theories about this issue are not conclusive, but children might experience increased lactose tolerance simply because they are consuming fewer dairy foods during this period of life than when they were babies. In any event, it is important to know your child's tolerance level for lactose because if he or she is able to consume some yogurt or milk or cheese, these will be an important added calcium source in the diet.

To easily test your child's tolerance level at home, simply be sure that your son or daughter ingests no lactose whatsoever for a period of about one week. Then give your child a small amount of a dairy food that has a naturally low lactose level. A good choice is an ounce of aged cheddar or swiss cheese. Give no other dairy foods or lactose during this time. If after twenty-four hours your child exhibits no symptoms of digestive distress, give two servings of aged cheese the next day. If symptoms occur during the following twenty-four hours, you will know that your child may be able to digest very small amounts of low-lactose foods and occasionally one-ounce servings of aged cheese may be included in your child's diet. If your child is able to tolerate lactose at this level, you may proceed to test other dairy foods. If your child reacts negatively to the cheese, he or she should probably avoid dairy foods entirely.

Next, test with yogurt, which is a valuable calcium source and is also available as a low-fat food. Choose only yogurt with live and active cultures. Give your child a half cup serving to try. If there are no symptoms, then offer your child one cup the next day. As always, if symptoms occur, withdraw the dairy product. If no symptoms occur, add this to the list of foods your child may be able to eat occasionally, or perhaps frequently, depending on his or her tolerance level. Work next with ice cream, followed by chocolate milk, and finally milk itself. Lactose-intolerant children have been known to tolerate many dairy foods in small amounts without any ill effects. To enhance your child's ability to digest some lactose without discomfort, studies have shown that digestibility is improved if the child follows these guidelines.

1. Eat small quantities of dairy foods throughout the day, rather than one large serving.

2. Eat dairy foods with other foods; this slows the action of digestion and allows whatever enzyme amount is present to act on the lactose for a longer period of time.

3. Eat the dairy food before a rest period when, again, the action of the gut is slowed.

4. Choose dairy foods containing chocolate. That's right, chocolate. Although it is not understood exactly why this is the case, studies have shown that chocolate milk is better tolerated by lactose-intolerant children than unflavored milk.

If your child seems to have some tolerance for dairy foods in small quantities, it is appropriate to try enzyme supplementation if you wish. You may pretreat milk at home with lactase enzyme drops or purchase pretreated milk in the store. As always, offer your child small quantities of these products, perhaps as little as a half cup at first, to try to ascertain his or her tolerance level. If you wish to try chewable enzyme supplements, refer to the manufacturer's directions. Usually, children will require three to five chewable lactase enzyme tablets before eating a dairy product, but again, this is a subjective issue. For best results, these tablets should be chewed up and swallowed just before your child eats the dairy food—not five minutes before, but immediately before. Chewing the enzyme supplements after eating will have no beneficial effect.

Challenging the Milk-Allergic Child

Parents will want to confer with their child's pediatrician or pediatric allergist with regard to the best way to challenge their child's food allergy. Basically, though, the intention is to recheck a child's allergic response to a known food allergen periodically to see whether or not the status of that child's allergy has changed. The reason challenge tests are not recommended for babies or very small children is that some allergic responses can get out of control and put these children in danger for their lives. Allergies are serious business, especially when the allergies are severe and the children are young. However, some children will have a decreased response to a known allergen as they grow and their immune system matures. Keeping tabs on which allergens affect your child, whether they are known or new, is important for planning your child's diet and monitoring his or her health.

One recognized method of challenge testing for the older child is often referred to as the single-food elimination diet. Under this plan, during a five-day period, the offending food is fed to the child on the first day, withdrawn for the next three days, and then given again on the fifth day. The principle is simple: If a particular food causes an allergic response, giving it to the child should elicit that response. Avoiding that food for the next several days will give the child a chance to recoup from the allergic reaction while, potentially, antibodies are being formed to fight the offending food the next time its constituents enter the bloodstream. On the fifth day, the child is challenged again with the offending food, and if an allergic response occurs, that particular food can be confirmed definitively as an allergen.

Most allergic reactions to food occur within an hour. But this is certainly not a rule. Many food reactions occur six to eight hours after the problem food is ingested. If your child reacts with inner ear fluid buildup or digestive distress, certainly these reactions can take longer than one hour to occur. Some foods affect children for as little as ten to fifteen minutes. Some children respond to an offending food with swollen lips that last about thirty minutes. Or a single itchy hive may develop on a cheek or earlobe and be gone within a few minutes. Some experts contend that allergies can cause bed-wetting at night or personality changes. One little girl I knew began each allergic reaction with a temper tantrum. Seemingly from out of nowhere, she would begin to cry and scream and carry on as if in the throes of a tantrum. But later, usually within an hour or two, she would begin to swell somewhere on her body, and more often than not, her mother would find hives or welts forming around a bug bite she had gotten earlier or scratches from plants she reacted to outdoors. These reactions may not be universal, but parents of allergic children should respect the wide range of allergic responses that can occur in people, many of which are valid, though perhaps as yet scientifically undocumented. Remember that while our current medical knowledge about immune responses is broad, it is still limited.

When looking for allergens, parents should note that the most common foods that cause reactions in children are milk, wheat, eggs, sugar, corn, food coloring, cocoa, peanuts, oranges, and preservatives. Many children also react negatively to caffeine found in tea, coffee, cola, and chocolate. If a child has several food sensitivities and only one problem food is removed from the diet, there may be little evidence of improvement. Therefore, when doing a food challenge, it is best to remove all forms of suspected allergens during the test period. That way you will not be confused by a reaction to egg, for instance, when you are looking for a reaction to milk.

The Rotary Diet

Allergic children who react negatively to several foods may be placed on a rotary diet by their pediatrician or allergist. This type of diet allows most foods to be eaten, but on a rotation basis, which allows little access to allergens. For example, a child may be able to have chicken on day one, beef on day two, lamb on day three, fish on day four, and so on. The pattern may be repeated, but the child will not be given chicken three days in a row. This ensures that the allergens he might be responding to in chicken are kept at a very low level. If he ate chicken three days in a row, there would be a build-up of allergens and antibodies in his blood, which could precipitate an immunological reaction.

In her books, *The Impossible Child* and *Is This Your Child?*, Dr. Doris J. Rapp, a board-certified environmental medical specialist, pediatric allergist, and clinical assistant professor of pediatrics at the State University of New York at Buffalo, carefully guides parents through the daily management of children with allergies. The latter work also addresses management of adults with allergies. Step by step, she outlines rotary diets and elimination diets. Her approach can help parents understand these feeding processes more fully and carry them out with success. Her books are also filled with case histories of allergic infants and children, which many parents will find interesting to study.

In an earlier work entitled *Allergies and Your Family*, published in 1980, Dr. Rapp lists possible foods associated with specific medical problems. She believes that children allergic to milk may exhibit some of the following symptoms: runny nose, wheezing and asthma, hyperactivity, eczema, hives, headache, ear problems, recurrent infections, bed-wetting, cystitis, muscle pain or weakness, joint tightness, colitis, duodenal ulcer, gall bladder disease, convulsions or tics, kidney problems, and high blood pressure. She also explains that many foods other than typical allergens naturally induce the release of histamine in the body causing hives or asthma, but this response is unrelated to the immunological allergic response. These foods are cheese, lobster, shrimp, mackerel, salmon, egg white, tomatoes, pork, chocolate, tuna, sausage, bananas, pineapple, papaya, and strawberries. Excess histamine may produce hives, flushing, nausea, diarrhea, and headaches.

Deflecting Feeding Problems

When I was a child, food and feeding were major family activities and were also elements of discipline. One of my mother's favorite punishments was to send the misbehaving child out on the back porch without food while the rest of the family was happily having dinner together. The misbehaving child then felt isolated, deprived, and guilty, not to mention hungry, although we were always given our meal when we repented. Other times, because I often ate slowly and was a fussy eater, mother sent me to another room to stand in the corner with my face to the wall. I learned how to become an expert at chewing my food into little bits and then sneakily spitting them out into my napkin, so it looked like I was eating, but actually I was swallowing nothing. Other friends have told me about their food avoidance escapades, which included hiding pancakes in dresser drawers, sneaking their dinner under the table to the dog, selling their school lunches, or swapping the whole apple for the whole bag of chocolate cookies.

The point is, kids do these things. They are not evil children and do not require capital punishment for fooling around with their food. But eating is important, especially when children require vital nutrients from foods they may not always adore. That's why it is imperative for parents of dairy-sensitive children to create a friendly feeding environment that is conducive to their children eating a variety of nutritious foods at home, at school, and while visiting friends or pursuing other outside activities.

The following is a list of suggestions for setting a positive tone for eating in your household. These are management techniques you can try to encourage your child to eat healthy foods and respect the role that food plays in his or her health. Some of these ideas may be difficult for some parents to accept, especially if they themselves were raised in a strict three-meal-a-day, no-snacking-in-between-meals, finish-everything-on-your-plate, eat-those-peas-or-no-dessert-for-you kind of atmosphere.

Great Feeding Idea #1   The first and most important rule is to forget the rules. There is no law requiring that eggs only be eaten at breakfast time and spaghetti only for lunch or dinner. Three meals a day may be appropriate in some cases, but children, and for that matter adults as well, need to eat several times a day, throughout the day, to keep their energy levels up. Especially if they have allergies, eating helps to keep the immune response supported by nutrients and functioning well at all times. The sky will not fall if your child has a sandwich before bedtime, his dinner directly after school and before baseball practice, a bowl of soup for breakfast, or consumes no cheese at all, ever. Healthy food choices are appropriate any time of the day or evening.

Great Feeding Idea #2   Teach your child that food is to be used for nutrition and energy. Children should be offered a variety of healthy choices and encouraged to try new foods. However they should not be punished or admonished for wanting to eat their favorites often, as long as their choices are nutritious. Teach your child that food is like the gas you put in the car. It will provide energy to help him or her get through the day and night. Teach your child that food will help him or her grow straight and strong like the flowers in the garden. When introducing new foods, remember that children who have been given the right of refusal tend to refuse less.

Great Feeding Idea #3   Help your child understand his or her food sensitivity. Teach your child that eating the wrong foods will make him or her sick or obese or will cause a headache. Give them the words to explain their condition to the baby-sitter, or to grandma, or to their day-care provider. Don't deny them dairy foods without an explanation, and give them the power to feel masterful over their sensitivity through knowledge about their condition. Encourage them to inquire, "Does this food have milk in it? I can't have any milk, it gives me a tummy ache."

Great Feeding Idea #4   Respect your child's ability to make choices about foods to eat. Let him help himself to appropriate foods when he needs a snack. Label the foods in the cupboard that are good choices for your child to make on his own. The key to success, however, is for parents to fill their cupboards with appropriate choices. It isn't fair to have three packages of cheesy chips in the pantry that mom and dad are going to eat, but that junior cannot. It isn't smart to have a half-gallon of gourmet ice cream in the freezer without also having a dairy-free ice cream alternative available for your five-year-old, unless you want to see a temper tantrum. Let your child help choose foods to buy at the supermarket, but do not put him in charge.

Great Feeding Idea #5   Enjoy mealtime with your child. Use this opportunity for socializing with friends, bonding as a family, and taking a few moments out of the chaos to eat together in a nonfrazzled atmosphere. No TV, no phone calls, no reading the paper. Sometimes lunch can be as short as ten minutes. But those ten minutes can be spent very well, talking together, sharing secrets, making plans.

Great Feeding Idea #6   Do not use food as a disciplinary tool. Don't make it an element of control. Children should not be denied food because they misbehaved or forced to eat foods they abhor as a punishment. Do not treat your children to foods they should not have as a means of rewarding them for something. Food should not be feared, revered, or exalted in importance beyond the reasonable.

Discipline your children in other ways. Not at the dinner table.

Great Feeding Idea #7   Set a good example. If you won't eat the broccoli, why should your child?

Great Feeding Idea #8   Understand that food guides are simply that—guides. Studies have shown that children, when given the opportunity to choose their own foods from a nutritious offering, will over the course of a day or several days naturally take in the proper amounts of calories and other nutrients they require. Do not turn the dinner table into a war zone. Put the right foods out on the table, and let the child eat. Balance their beverages with food so that they are not filling up on apple juice or formula before sitting down to mealtime with the family. Remember that water is a nice drink, too.

Great Feeding Idea #9   Stock your freezer and your cupboards with dairy-free food choices and foods that are easy for your child to eat on quick notice. If necessary, prepare individual servings for the freezer that can be warmed up in no time in the microwave oven. Let your child help you in the kitchen; this will stimulate his or her interest in food and the way it is prepared. One of my favorite friends is severely lactose intolerant. When we go to a party, he always sticks very close to me and eats only what I eat. The reason is because even at forty-seven years old, he has no clue about how foods are prepared or what ingredients are in which foods. If your child works with you in the kitchen, he or she learns that baked potatoes have no milk and that broiled chicken with cherry sauce has no milk, and that stir-fried beef and broccoli is milk-free.

Great Feeding Idea #10   Understand that many small children seem to be vegetarians naturally—they simply don't like meat. Rather than fretting or fighting, take a positive step and learn more about vegetarianism. Learn which foods your child should be eating in place of meat and offer those. If you wish, try meat again later. If you insist that your child eat meat, but the only meat he will eat is a burger from a fast-food restaurant, treat him to the burger once in a while. There are some healthy choices out there, too.

Great Feeding Idea #11 Expect that toddlers and small children will make a mess. Feeding themselves independently of you is more important than the kitchen floor. To help avoid the mess, give them small, manageable quantities rather than a platefull of food all at once. Make bath time an activity after the dairy-free pudding has been served. Recognize that if your child is writing on the wall with the ketchup, she is probably not hungry and needs to get out of her high chair.

Great Feeding Idea #12 Help your child make independent, but appropriate, choices by only offering two healthy alternatives. Perhaps your child can choose between an egg or oatmeal, between carrots or peas, mashed potatoes or baked beans. Don't open up the full realm of possibility with every meal. Children are overwhelmed by vast choices.

Great Feeding Idea #13 Get help. Consult a registered dietitian who can construct an individualized meal plan for your child that is appropriate for his or her age and food sensitivities.

Great Feeding Idea #14 Don't take it personally. If your child won't eat a dish you have worked hard to prepare, just enjoy the meal for yourself. Most children, even small ones, are capable of preparing a peanut-butter-and-jelly sandwich in lieu of the new dish or can be satisfied by eating the other foods at the table. Don't be offended. Move on.

Feeding Your Child During Adolescence

The title of this section is really an oxymoron. No parent feeds his or her child during adolescence and the later teen years. Children ages eleven through eighteen are pretty much on their own when it comes to eating. They eat lunch in school, meet their friends at the mall for a burger, order pizza on Saturday nights, and attend school functions and parties where food is a definite part of the activity. Still, there are a few things parents can do to help ensure that their children are receiving the nutrients they need. After all, these are very important years, health-wise, because girls and boys are going through substantial growth spurts and are being challenged by fluctuating hormonal levels.

During this time, adolescents and teens are often extremely busy, are prone to many illnesses, and function on erratic schedules where studying, practicing sports, and partying often take precedence over sleeping and eating right. This is also a time of experimentation, when boys and girls often have their first encounter with tobacco, alcohol, or drugs. Teenagers who continue to use these substances will surely be compromising their health, if not their lives. Therefore, the health management role parents can play during this time is a very vital one, but one probably best played out subtly in the background.

One of the most important things parents can do for their young teenagers is to help supply them with the nutrients their bodies require to sustain their rapid growth and development. Where your child's bones are concerned, these are peak years for calcium storage, and for girls, especially, adequate calcium consumption is essential to help reduce the risk of debilitating osteoporosis after menopause. If your teen is eating a steady diet of burgers and fries, it may be essential to give him or her a daily vitamin and calcium supplement. Studies show that calcium intake during this period is, for many teens, very low. Lots of meals at the local fast-food restaurant simply will not supply your child with the nutrients he or she needs.

It is also very helpful for parents to stock the refrigerator and cupboards at home with nutritious foods and snacks. Kids are hungry at all hours of the day and night, and they will help themselves to foods that are beneficial to their overall health if there are good choices awaiting them in the kitchen at home. Face it, you cannot be sure what your teens are eating away from home, but you do have some control over the foods they consume while they are at home. Be sure and have on hand a variety of fresh fruits and healthful foods that can be grabbed quickly from the refrigerator. Good choices include tuna salad, salmon salad, and cut-up vegetables and a healthy dip, perhaps one made from soft tofu blended with dry soup mix or other spices. Always stock the refrigerator with calcium-fortified juice and fruit drinks. They are better than soda any day. Or show your son or daughter how to make a cooler out of a half-and-half mixture of calcium-fortified orange juice and fruit-flavored carbonated water. Set a good example by leaving the chips on the store shelves and instead choosing lower-fat snack foods such as popcorn and pretzels. Prepare a blend of fortified cereals mixed with mini-pretzels and milk-free semisweet chocolate morsels and raisins in a large bowl for quick and easy snacking.

Give your dairy-sensitive teen the nutrition information he or she needs to make decisions on his or her own about foods to choose when eating in restaurants or at school. Find out what's on the school lunch menu and recommend dairy-free foods your child can select. Find out which restaurants the gang likes to frequent, and learn what is on the menus there. Help your son or daughter make his or her own healthy choices. Did you know that all the pizza chains across America will make pizza without cheese? Cheese-free pizza provides your teen with the opportunity to eat what all the other kids are eating, but without getting sick.

Adolescent and teenage boys should be eating between 2,800 and 3,000 calories per day. Their diet should include about 1,200 mg calcium per day, along with substantial amounts of vitamins A, D, E, phosphorus, and iron. They should be eating about eleven servings from the grain group; five servings from the vegetable group; four servings from the fruit group; seven servings from the protein group; and the nutritional equivalent of two to three cups of milk. Ideally, your teenage son has developed some pretty good eating habits because of your attention to his diet since infancy, but even so, he is likely to be fatigued, anxious, and under stress often enough to sabotage even the best diet at times.

Your daughter between the ages of eleven and eighteen is undergoing some remarkable changes as well. To sustain her growth and development, she should be eating about 2,200 calories per day and as much as 2,800 calories per day if she is highly active in sports. Normally, girls of this age should be eating about nine servings from the grain group; four servings from the vegetable group; three servings from the fruit group; six servings from the protein group; and the nutritional equivalent of two to three cups of milk. Some experts believe that teenage girls need to take in at least 1,200 mg of calcium a day, which is closer to the nutritional equivalent of four cups of milk. Government studies have shown that only 63 percent of teenage girls receive the recommended daily allowance for calcium. Yet, it is known that girls need to store substantial amounts of calcium in preparation for the substantial bone loss they will experience after menopause when their estrogen levels plummet. Teenage girls who cannot eat dairy foods must be given calcium-rich alternative foods or supplements to ensure their good health now and later.

5 Feeding Your Child at School or Day Care

In 1991, about 60 percent of all mothers with children younger than six years old were in the labor force. This compares with 40 percent in 1970 and accounts for almost 9.6 million working women with preschool-aged children today. Currently, about 75 percent of women with children ages six to seventeen are in the work force compared to about 58 percent twenty years ago. That correlates to an estimated 11.1 million children younger than six and 25.8 million children ages six to seventeen whose mothers are currently in the work force.

During the past ten years, the single most significant shift in caring for these children has been away from in-home care and into day-care centers or nursery schools. Generally, women who work full-time tend to use day-care centers, while those who work part-time are most likely to utilize in-home care. What this means is that millions of children who are dairy sensitive are not eating all of their meals and snacks at home, even if they are as young as one or two years old. Certainly if your infant is in a day-care setting, he or she will be drinking the formula you provide. Or, if you are a breast-feeding mother, your baby may be given expressed milk that you have bottled or frozen beforehand. In either case, feeding the dairy-sensitive infant away from home is a fairly easy procedure.

The preschool or school-aged child, however, does offer some challenges. Parents of dairy-sensitive children will always have an obligation to oversee their children's food choices to some degree, especially when the children are in school or in a day-care center. For some children, the out-of-home eating situation may occur soon after their birth, and for others, a little later in their lives. But eventually all children will be eating meals and snacks in school. This may last from the time they are at least five years old until they are twenty-one years old and having meals in college dorms. As parents, you will be intervening somewhat in the school or day-care setting all along the way. You will be consulting with either the caregiver or the teacher or the administrator or the food-service director. Parents will continue to be a link between their children and the children's food for many years, and in some situations will even have to advocate heavily for their children's welfare.

Parents wear many hats in the out-of-home feeding situation. They serve as experts, giving information about milk-protein allergy or lactose intolerance to their child's teacher or day-care provider. To help the professional understand your child's condition, it might be a good idea for you to type up a short fact sheet to which the professional might refer from time to time. The fact sheet should include your child's name, your name and phone number, a physician's phone number, the name of your child's specific medical problem, a brief explanation of the nature of the problem, a list of foods your child may not have, a list of foods your child may have, along with information about what you are willing to do to help your child in the day-care or school setting. You may even need to list emergency information for children with severe allergies, or supply the professional with medications appropriate for your child.

Parents of dairy-sensitive children will also be providers of special foods for their children or may act as teacher aids in a number of settings. In the fact sheet you prepare, you might list foods that you will be willing to supply to the school or day-care center for your child. For example, you could send dairy-free cupcakes, which could be stored in the school's freezer and given to your child when other children have cupcake treats. Or you might want to provide the day-care center or school with calcium-fortified juice for your child to drink instead of the regular beverage served. Many parents offer to be room mothers or room fathers and volunteer to bring all the snacks and treats for all the children. By doing this, you can ensure that your child will only be having dairy-free snacks and treats because you will be in charge of bringing them.

There are other ways for parents to be helpful in the school or day-care situation. You may wish to volunteer to be a chaperon on school trips, which will let you help your child eat an appropriate lunch in a restaurant along the way. Or you could volunteer to act as an aide in the classroom or day-care center for special events, thereby being able to keep a close eye on the food your child is being offered. This may be especially useful if other parents are supplying the snacks or treats for holiday celebrations. You could also provide your child with a snack or meal packed at home for all eating situations, whether in the classroom or on a field trip. Make sure that he or she has an extra special lunch bag or box, so this difference becomes something to be proud of in front of the other children. Helping your child eat properly while not at home allows him to feel as good as possible physically and encourages him to respect the importance of his dairy sensitivity. Your extra effort will help him to eat well and feel supported and loved by you even when you aren't around.

Parents may play the role of advocate for their child as well. This is especially true for parents of school-aged children. In the school setting, children may be given milk during snack time in kindergarten or as part of the school breakfast or lunch programs. Children may not be offered juice alternatives until they reach middle school or junior high, where typically, more food choices are offered during the school lunch period. Some children won't be given much choice until they reach high school. In these situations, parents will have to advocate for their child, working as cooperatively as possible with school administrators and food-service directors to provide alternatives for their children who cannot drink milk or eat other dairy foods.

But what can parents rightfully expect from their child's school or day-care provider? Well, that depends. Just the other day, I read about a five-year-old boy whose parents claim he was dismissed from the private school he attended in New York because he had a peanut allergy. They contend that the school's administrator was unwilling to provide separate snacks or meals for this child and insinuated that because of his allergy, he would not fit in with the other children, who were capable of eating any food. Now, if this is indeed what happened, has the private school done anything illegal? Can the parents demand that their child be readmitted to the school and that the school make certain accommodations for the fact that this child cannot have peanuts or any food derived from peanuts including peanut oil and peanut butter? The resolution to this situation has yet to be determined legally in the state of New York. But the outcome of the litigation, if there is a lawsuit filed, will be watched by many parents of allergic children across the nation as well as by school officials.

While there are federal laws and guidelines governing public schools and private schools, interpretations of these laws may differ or clash with the laws and guidelines of individual states. There are no clear-cut answers to the problems raised by allergic and lactose-intolerant children in school or day-care settings as yet. Some day-care providers are very willing to accommodate milk allergic or lactose-intolerant children, often with a little help from parents. Likewise, some private schools will do the same. Similarly, some public schools do provide accommodation for children with food allergies or intolerances, while others clearly do not. And while there seems to be substantial legal ground on which to base a case for your child's receiving accommodation, in many situations, there are gray areas, and the laws have not been fully tested.

According to the *School Safety Handbook*, 1986, compiled by the Association of School Business Officials International in Reston, Virginia, and the National Safety Council, "When legislation made public school attendance mandatory for children up to a certain age, it brought with it certain inescapable obligations. Since school attendance is mandatory in the United States, schools are required to provide pupils with a safe and healthful environment." Some believe that laws meant to provide protection for people with handicaps also apply to children with allergies and/or food intolerances. Specifically, Section 504 of the Rehabilitation Act of 1973 states, "No otherwise qualified individual with handicaps in the United States . . . shall, solely by reason of his handicap, be excluded from the participation in, be denied the benefits of, or be subjected to discrimination under any program or activity receiving Federal financial assistance. . . ." In fact, several regulations for the implementation of Section 504 require schools to safeguard parents' rights, to make sure that the needs of a child with a handicap are met fairly and appropriately, and to act in partnership with parents for the welfare of the child.

Many school officials act on the presumption that Section 504 only refers to children who are in special education programs. But Section 504 rulings clearly indicate that schools must provide related services and accommodations to "handicapped students" in regular classrooms also. The interpretation of the word "handicapped" is recognized by most experts in the field to mean any physical or mental disorder or condition affecting one or more body systems that substantially limits one or more major life activity including breathing and other activities such as walking, speaking, or eating. According to this definition, food allergies and intolerances absolutely are included in the definition of "handicapped," and public schools subject to the law, along with other schools or institutions receiving federal funds, therefore are required to provide accommodation to the child with food allergies or intolerances. What this means, then, is that your dairy-sensitive child has the right to eat in school without consuming foods that would jeopardize his or her health. He or she cannot be forced to drink milk with lunch or eat a grilled cheese sandwich.

This statute was recently bolstered by the passage of the Americans with Disabilities Act. Borrowing from Section 504 of the Rehabilitation Act of 1973, the ADA extends many rights to individuals with disabilities in public places such as restaurants, hotels, theaters, stores, doctor's offices, museums, private schools, and child-care programs. Children with allergies or asthma are generally recognized as having "impairments," which do qualify them for some accommodation when appropriate, even if their allergies or asthma are controlled by medication. According to Ellie Goldberg, M.Ed., an educational rights specialist with expertise in the area of allergic children's rights, "A private preschool cannot refuse to enroll children because giving medication or adapting snacks for students with allergies requires staff training or because insurance rates might go up."

If this proves to be unequivocal, our little boy with the peanut allergy will be readmitted to the private New York preschool. Clearly, your dairy-sensitive child does have rights in school settings. But how real are those rights? Legal experts maintain that rights remain theoretical until someone asserts them. According to *A Handbook on Legal Rights of Disabled People in Massachusetts* by Robert Crabtree, Lawrence Kotin, and Nancy Rich, asserting one's rights "often requires patience, persuasiveness, resourcefulness and expert assistance. Although it is often frustrating and discouraging to go through the process of arguing for your rights, it is important to remember that it is through this process that rights are secured and passed on to future generations."

Goldberg advises parents to work cooperatively but firmly with school personnel to provide a supportive environment for their children with allergies. She has written that "Parents of 'other health-impaired' students can work with the school to create an Individualized Education Plan (IEP). An IEP is a formal written agreement that documents the special needs of the student with food allergies." Parents, teachers, and administrators can work together to develop an IEP, which would spell out specific guidelines for the classroom teachers, for handling special events such as class parties, lunch, and field trips, and for an emergency plan. This type of procedure is especially important for children with allergies severe enough to cause asthma or life-threatening anaphylaxis. The IEP could give general information about allergies and allergic reactions. Parents could also instruct teachers and administrators about the proper use of the emergency adrenaline injection their child might need to have on hand, and could likewise include this information in the IEP.

In a publication entitled *Food Allergy News,* published in August/September 1992, Goldberg asserts that the United States Department of Agriculture Regulations "require federally funded school breakfast, snack, and lunch programs to provide special meals or menu substitutions at no extra charge to children who have a physician's documentation of 1) the student's medical or other special diet restriction and 2) which food or ingredients are to be omitted from the child's menu and which food choices or ingredients may be substituted." She explains that the USDA regulations require cafeteria staff to provide parents with a listing of ingredients used in lunch or breakfast meals.

Despite this, parents of dairy-sensitive children may face some difficult times when dealing with their child's eating situation in school. Laws are often controversial, and the interpretation of this one is also potentially volatile, considering the power of school administrators to set regulations within their own district and the fact that parents, although they may advocate for their children, are not necessarily recognized authorities on the subject of legal rights for children. The Food and Nutrition Information Center of the United States Department of Agriculture is a storehouse of information regarding this and other related issues and can provide parents with helpful information. A USDA publication from the Food and Nutrition Service division states:

> Schools shall make substitutions in foods listed in this section for students who are considered handicapped under 7 CFR part 15b and whose handicap restricts their diet. Schools may also make substitutions for nonhandicapped students who are unable to consume the regular lunch because of medical or other special dietary needs. Substitutions shall be made on a case by case basis only when supported by a statement of the need for substitutions that includes recommended alternate foods, unless otherwise exempted by FNS. Such statement shall, in the case of a handicapped student, be signed by a physician or, in the case of a nonhandicapped student, by a recognized medical authority.

Cecilia Rokusek, Ed.D., R.D., CHE, Assistant to the Vice President for Health Affairs, and professor, Department of Family Medicine and Dental Hygiene at the University of South Dakota School of Medicine, however, cautions parents about the strict implementation of these regulations. She points to a USDA Food and Nutrition Service Instruction 783-2, Rev. 1, which states that "food service personnel are not to make the determination of whether a child is handicapped." The instruction also states that "generally, children with food allergies or intolerances are *not* handicapped." Rokusek reminds parents that special diets are a relatively new area in child nutrition programs, and specific steps should be undertaken when parents seek to secure food accommodations for their children.

Rokusek recommends the following plan to parents of children on restricted diets:

1. A request for a special diet should be accompanied by a physician's order.

2. The special diet request should contain specific language for required food substitutions, when possible.

3. School menus may be submitted to the physician who could then request specific deletions of food items. A registered dietitian may help with this. Ingredient labels may also be provided for scrutiny by the health professional.

4. A school nurse may provide the service to the school, although approval of the nurse's recommendations in writing from the physician should still be obtained.

5. If substitutions offered by the school food service are approved, implementation may begin.

6. If the substitutions offered by the school food service are not accepted, the food-service director should be referred to the physician or other health professional for consultation.

7. Some substitutions may involve expense that the school food service cannot underwrite. Alternative funding sources will need to be secured.

8. When all of these issues have been resolved, the individual-ized program can be implemented.

Many schools will accept the authority of a registered nurse or physician's assistant in helping formulate an appropriate food program for the child with food allergies or intolerances. But most importantly, parents need to work cooperatively with the school board, school administration, and food-service personnel in order to accomplish their goals.

In a paper written by M. Ricci in the April 1991 publication *American School Food Service Association* (Vol. 45, pp. 69–70), the author states that even though the meal pattern in school lunch programs is very specific, schools are required to make food sub-stitutions where necessary to accommodate a medical or special dietary need. Handicapped or chronically ill students must be served meals that meet their needs and still qualify for re-imbursement. The author goes on to state, "The needs of students with food allergies and those with religious dietary re-strictions also must be respected." Ricci adds that the most com-mon request is for a substitution for the "fluid milk component."

Note the difference in language the author uses. When de-scribing substitutions made for handicapped or chronically ill students, the implication is that substitutions *must* be made, while food-allergic children or lactose-intolerant children should have their needs "respected." Is a child with a milk allergy or lactose intolerance in the same category as a child who is "chronically ill," say with diabetes? Is a child with asthma in the same category as a child with cystic fibrosis? These are some of the determinations that may have to be made in your child's case if you believe special accommodation should be provided by your child's school.

Who should pay for substitutions in the school lunch menu? Clearly, the school district will be responsible in some cases, if your child has multiple handicaps, for example. In other situations, parents may be asked to provide a food component that may not be easily accessible to the school. In the case of a milk-protein-allergic child, that substitution might be a calcium-fortified soy beverage, for example, which is not available to the school personnel through their regular vendors. If it is determined that your child will be permitted substitutions, and the school meals program is unable to absorb the cost of the special diet food items, there are several other places to look for funding. These include a payment from the school itself, Medicaid, private insurance, state programs for children with special health-care needs, special or established state department programs, private payment, Social Security Supplemental Income (SSI), and the Women, Infant, and Children Supplemental Feeding Program (WIC).

In pursuing this, parents may come face to face with a number of barriers for establishing their child's individualized feeding program in school. For one, school professionals may lack the training in implementing special dietary programs, or some school professionals may fail to recognize the significance of nutrition and therefore deem your requests to be trivial. Parents with real concerns in this area may need to put together an advocacy team for their child consisting of outside professionals, such as a registered dietitian, their child's pediatrician or allergist, and perhaps an emissary from a federal agency such as the National School Lunch Program, to work with the food-service professionals in the school setting.

Critical issues in school often go beyond food. Especially for highly allergic children or children with asthma, there are the issues of emergency management, daily management, and medication as well. Goldberg, as a representative of Mothers of Asthmatics, Inc. in Newton, Massachusetts, describes the situations experienced by two different asthmatic children in two different schools and focuses on the variations in their management.

> Doug wakes up cranky after a night interrupted by several wheezing episodes. After his morning medications, his breathing seems almost normal. His mother, due at work by nine, feels he can make it through the day if the teachers let him take it easy and

give him his medication on time. His mother alerts the school nurse and teachers to Doug's condition and goes off to work confident that they know what to do.

Goldberg explains that Doug is in a school willing to adapt to his medical needs and the nurse and teacher have participated in the formulation of Doug's IEP, or Individualized Education Plan. Doug, depending upon how he feels during the school day, may be excused from vigorous gym activities or may be allowed temporary adjustments to his time spent outdoors. He may also be given his medication as required. In contrast, Goldberg describes the case of Beth, whose asthmatic condition is treated much differently at her school.

> Two days after a severe asthma episode, Beth feels better and has stopped wheezing. Her mother takes Beth to school with her additional medication and requests that she be allowed to avoid outdoor play during the cold weather. The school nurse is not there to discuss Beth's medication. The classroom teacher responds, "The school policy is that if a child is well enough to come to school, then she is well enough to go outside."

Beth went home with her mother. Beth's school did not allow any adaptation of her participation in school activities that day. Goldberg asserts that children with asthma and allergies should not be barred from participating fully in school, and that they are legally entitled to receive accommodation for their conditions. She believes that schools should not send children home or exclude them from field trips and other activities, but rather, should provide access to prescribed medications, which might make their participation possible. Schools should "allow for temporary adjustments for students who might require some restrictions on vigorous gym, sports or outdoor play, especially in cold weather."

These cases typify some of the predicaments often encountered by parents of dairy-sensitive children in school. Children should not be barred from drinking orange juice instead of milk or from bringing a dairy-free lunch when a dairy meal is being served. Parents of dairy-sensitive children should be given the opportunity to work with the food-service director, who should cooperatively manage to make substitutions for milk-protein-allergic or lactose-intolerant children. Children must be permitted to take lactase enzyme tablets before eating dairy foods if this method is appropriate for their complete digestion. In particular, however, the details of how to accomplish these goals will depend upon the successful advocacy of parents. Personally, I am not an expert in this area. If you require more information on this topic, please contact the following experts for help:

Ellie Goldberg, M.Ed.
Educational Rights Specialist
79 Elmore St.
Newton, MA 02159
617-965-9637

The National Information Center for Children
    and Youth with Handicaps
PO Box 1492
Washington, DC 20013
800-999-5599

U.S. Department of Education
Office for Civil Rights
Washington, DC 20202-1328

Center for Law and Education
955 Massachusetts Ave.
Cambridge, MA 02139

The National Committee for Citizens in Education
900 Second St. NE, Suite 8
Washington, DC 20002
202-408-0447

The Child Care Law Center
22 Second St., Fifth Floor
San Francisco, CA 94105
415-495-5498

Office on the Americans with Disabilities Act
Civil Rights Division
U.S. Department of Justice
PO Box 66118
Washington, DC 20035-6118

Parent Information Center
Peer and Family Training Network Project on the ADA
PO Box 1422
Concord, NH 03302-1422
603-224-0402

Educational Rights of Child with Disabilities:
A Primer for Advocates
Eileen Ordover and Kathleen B. Boundy
Center for Law and Education
955 Massachusetts Ave.
Cambridge, MA 02139
617-876-6611

U. S. Department of Agriculture
Food and Nutrition Information Center
National Agricultural Library
Beltsville, MD 20705-2351

Allergy and Asthma Network/Mothers of Asthmatics, Inc.
3554 Chain Bridge Rd., Suite 200
Fairfax, VA 22030
703-385-4403
800-878-4403

Solving Emotional Conflicts at School

Today, many more children are diagnosed with food allergies
than may have been in past years because members of medical

fields have come to recognize and accept the significance of these allergies. Yet there are still some educators, administrators, and child-care providers who believe that allergies are "all in the head." One woman I know, an intelligent, active, woman in the local community center, once told me that asthma was a child's way of calling for his mother's attention. She truly believed that in 1995, the way to treat asthma was to send all working women home. Even though we know today that asthma is a disease of the immune system, many people, even people in professional child-care settings, consider allergies and asthma a sign of a child's poor emotional development: If he has allergies, he has psychological problems.

You and your children know that this is simply not so. Certainly, food allergies can cause symptoms that affect a child's behavior. This is undeniable in medicine today. And certainly children who struggle with allergic reactions can develop fluctuations in their responses to the stressful situations they encounter every day, all day long, during play or while in school. Allergies cause children to have physiological reactions that may make them ill or cranky or angry or despondent or tired. Allergic children may have very high highs and very low lows. The same may be true of children with food intolerances. They simply are made unwell by the digestive distress they experience and by the interruption of nutrients flowing through their blood to their muscles, nerves, and brain. Some so-called normal kids have ups and downs too, but children with allergies and intolerances are often children with highly sensitive physiological systems, who may appear more emotional or more reactive than the others.

Teachers' comments can hurt children. Teachers wield enormous power over children, especially young children who believe everything their teachers may say. Teachers are capable of making children feel hurt, shame, fright, frustration, and anger. Teachers who are suspicious of a child, especially an allergic child, may even unconsciously contribute to that child's loss of self-confidence and self-esteem. Children who are maligned at school by teachers, aides, or other children, carry the hurt with them for many years, often into adulthood.

And everyone knows that kids who are different in some way receive more than their fair share of negative responses. If your child wheezes or itches or has eczema or has frequent diarrhea or vomits in school or needs to eat special food or take special medicine, he or she needs to be in a school setting that is being watched over by a sensitive teacher and educational community. I believe that it is your job as parents of such a child to monitor the comments of teachers and students in the classroom from time to time and be prepared to step in, if necessary, to spare your child from intimidation, should it be forthcoming.

Communicate actively with your child. Reserve a special time each day for quiet conversation, just between the two of you. Without other distractions, your child may be extremely willing to chat with you about his or her day, and the good and bad experiences that occurred. Don't be judgmental. Give your child the opportunity to speak freely, to say what's on his or her mind. During that time, don't put your own value judgments on the child's comments. You might start the conversation by asking, "What was the best thing that happened to you today?" Then you could ask, "What was the worst thing that happened to you today?" Check periodically to make sure that your child understands the scope of his or her allergies or intolerances. Help your child understand what is happening in his or her body, and offer support for the feelings he or she may be encountering. Dairy-sensitive children are bound to have feelings of anger, frustration, and embarrassment. Reassure your child that you understand how she feels, and that you will always do whatever you can to help her cope.

Give your child the words to say when he or she is being maligned. Instruct your child to speak out for herself, and to tell the other students that making fun of her is a cruel and rude thing to do. Even a four-year-old can be taught to say, "Please stop saying those things to me, they hurt my feelings." An older child should be able to respond by saying something like, "I am upset right now because my allergies are bothering me. I'll feel better after I take some medicine." Or, "I understand that many people don't know much about lactose intolerance, but if you have any questions I will be happy to answer them."

Your child will need to learn how to recognize when his allergies or intolerances are interfering with his ability to function well in the classroom setting. If your allergic child has frequent temper tantrums and requires a time-out to recoup, give him the opportunity to separate, relax, and rejuvenate, so that he can resume his activities in an acceptable manner. When he is calm, you can explain to him that his allergies might be contributing to his behavior and that taking some medication or eating properly during the rest of the day might help him feel, and therefore act, better.

Twenty-five years ago, before time-out was invented as a proven parenting strategy, my oldest son often had difficulty controlling himself in class when he was in elementary school. This was due to a combination of factors, but his highly reactive allergic responses were certainly contributory. I did not want him to disrupt the class or be disrespectful to the teacher, and I certainly did not want the teacher to become so angry with my son that she would lose her head and make demeaning remarks to him which could have serious consequences. So, each semester when he was placed with a new teacher, I made it a point to speak to the teacher and request that he be sent out of the room for a few minutes to cool off whenever she felt it necessary. Of course, this gave the teacher the opportunity to cool off, too. I cannot tell you how many times I walked into the school during the day as a volunteer to hear my son call to me from down the hall, "Hi Mom. I'm just sitting out here for a little while!" By the way, he grew up to graduate from high school with honors and is now a high-school math teacher who also attends graduate school. Apparently his being sent out of the classroom at least several times a week did not have a negative impact on his education.

Other parents may have some very valuable advice for you if your family is experiencing difficulties in a school setting. Speak to other parents of allergic children through support groups or a local parents organization. Request parent-teacher conferences to stay up to date with your child's school experience. Recognize that some people, even teachers and other child-care professionals, are uninformed about allergies and food intolerances. Offer them your expertise. Perhaps your child's pediatric allergist could address a PTA meeting or provide a teachers' workshop. Do what you can to help those with deeply ingrained biases become informed so that stereotypical images and misconceptions can be eliminated from their attitudes. Enlist the help of school administrators or school-board members when appropriate. Encourage school personnel to come to you with their questions.

Missing School

It is very likely that your child with food allergies and intolerances will miss school occasionally, perhaps more frequently than other children. You must accept this and support your child in his or her efforts to keep up scholastically and maintain social contact with the other children in class. It may be hard to do at times, but parents must not blame their children for being ill and must learn to respect their children's need for rest and recuperation. Especially after a serious episode of wheezing, vomiting, hives, or diarrhea, the body needs time to recoup its energy stores and stabilize itself.

Usually, a few missed days here and there will not affect a child's performance in school or his or her relationships with friends. But sometimes, missing school will result in a child's falling behind in the work or becoming estranged with the other children. In all cases, schools have specific policies regarding homework and absences, and parents should make themselves aware of what these policies are. Schools also may have policies regarding the participation of children upon their immediate return to school. Will your child be expected to fully participate in vigorous gym activities or athletic programs? How will your child be singled out if he or she misses several days of school? Will he or she be denied the opportunity to try out for the school play or go on a field trip? How will your child be tutored if he or she misses several days of school? Will the teacher allow extra time to make up a test or turn in a paper? Who will administer medication should it be necessary upon your child's return to school? Is there a nurse on staff, or will parents be expected to drop in to give medication? Is a physician's note required? How will your child's grades be affected by the policies currently in place?

Some flexibility is essential when managing children who miss several days of school. In the best cases, your child's educational setting will be supportive of your desire for your child to achieve and participate as fully as possible, despite the possibility of absences. Parents and teachers who communicate well with each other are much more successful in managing the children in their charge. Working together in an atmosphere of mutual respect yields the best results for everyone involved, especially the children.

Remember that allergies and intolerances are not contagious diseases. Your child, though ill, may still see friends at home or speak on the phone to keep in contact with buddies. If your child is going to be absent frequently, it might be a good idea to purchase an extra set of textbooks to keep at home. This makes it easier for the child to stay current in class. Set up a tutoring schedule, if necessary, with either a professional tutor or another child from the same class.

Make sure that notices from school about upcoming events or program deadlines, the school newspaper, and reminders from teachers or coaches get sent home or are made available for you to pick up from school. Maintain a good relationship with the school secretary or principal's administrative assistant. This person is very knowledgeable about all aspects of the school setting, curricular and extracurricular, and will be an invaluable resource to you. Has your child's class been shown a video that is available for you to rent and bring home for your child to watch? Has your child made a drawing or completed a book report that can be taken to school for the class bulletin board? There is much parents can do to help children maintain their standing in school and their social relationships there. I've touched on only a handful of ideas for parents to explore.

6 | Kids' McMeals in Restaurants

Everyone deserves a break today! Let's face it. Eating out in restaurants is as American as Chicken McNuggets, which, incidentally, your dairy-sensitive child might not be able to eat. Kids love those little meals in little bags with little servings and little drinks and little toys—what a concept! They're great fun for children and their parents. Those special meals offered in fast-food restaurants will soon be a part of your life, if they aren't already. No, they may not be nutritionally equivalent to fresh salmon with steamed broccoli, but your child will be eating fast food and enjoying the experience immensely.

Eating in Fast-Food Restaurants

Fast-food restaurants harbor both good and bad foods. Just as there are some nutritional disasters lurking there, there are some healthy choices available for your child and some milk-free choices as well. You may have to do a little detective work, but all fast-food restaurants offer something for the dairy-sensitive child. Also, in response to consumer demand, fast-food chains can now provide you with a complete list of menu items and their ingredients. Ask for these brochures when you stop in to the local large chain restaurants. They will help you make appropriate food choices for your child.

Be aware that milk and its by-products can sometimes pop up in the weirdest places. I have been told that some fast-food french fries are laced with a lactose coating, and that the new broasted chicken restaurants inject milk by-product solutions into the meat to make it sweet and juicy. Can you imagine why whey would show up in taco meat? Neither can I. But it very well might be there. Many large chains provide their franchise stores with food and ingredients. But sometimes franchise owners use local suppliers for some menu items, such as buns and salad dressing. Therefore, no blanket recommendations can be made regarding milk-free foods in fast-food restaurants. Rather, you will have to spend a few moments with the manager of the local restaurants your children frequent. The best time to do this is late in the afternoon, after the lunch crowd has gone, and the dinner hour hasn't yet begun.

Here are a few general guidelines to help you select milk-free foods for your child in a fast-food restaurant:

1. Avoid any breaded product such as fried chicken, chicken nuggets, fingers, tenders, etc. as well as fish sticks, filets, and the like. Dried milk is almost always an ingredient in bread coating mixes.

2. Skip the cheese products. No cheeseburgers, grilled chicken and cheese sandwiches, salads with shredded cheese, or seafaring specialties, which are usually breaded fish patties with cheese melted on top.

3. Skip the basic milk foods such as shakes, ice-cream desserts, sour-cream toppers, and macaroni and cheese.

4. Watch out for special sauces. Many of them are buttermilk based. The mildly lactose-intolerant child may be able to tolerate some buttermilk, but it is not suitable for the moderately intolerant or milk-protein-allergic child.

5. Select salad dressings from the oil/vinegar varieties such as Italian and vinaigrette. The red French dressings should be fine, as should the Thousand Island dressing and others made from a mayonnaise base.

6. Choose the plainest food possible. Select a grilled chicken sandwich without sauce. Select a hamburger (ketchup, mustard, onion, and pickle are fine). Order a taco without the

cheese or sour cream, but guacamole should be okay, and salsa is definitely okay.

7. Salad bars are usually good choices. Skip the macaroni or potato salad, though. There may be milk in the dressing. Gelatin salads that are not white are safe. Even some of them that are white are safe, thanks to a variety of artificial ingredients, but to be very sure, select only the clear gelatin salads.

8. Ask about the buns. Some of them contain milk or whey. They may be fine for the lactose-intolerant child because the amount of lactose in a little bun is probably very small, but they may be inappropriate for the milk-protein-allergic child, unless you are certain of his or her allergic threshold.

9. Potato bars are great. A baked potato topped with chili or salsa is a terrific treat. You don't even need dairy-free margarine, which incidentally, is often available at fast-food restaurants. Skip the sour cream and cheesy broccoli toppings.

10. Enjoy the nacho chips, but not the cheese. Dip your chips in guacamole or salsa or chili or spaghetti sauce. They make great scoopers for Spanish rice.

11. At breakfast, your child can probably enjoy bacon and eggs, especially if the eggs are sunny-side up. Scrambled eggs may contain milk. Check to be sure. The bacon is okay, and so is the toasted bagel. Of course, you do know that biscuits are all made with milk, as are croissants, and those wonderful cinnamon buns. Avoid the French toast, pancakes, and waffles. They are all made with milk. Your child will have to enjoy these treats at home, where they can be made milk-free.

12. Skip the desserts, too, unless you can read the ingredients somewhere. I would be suspicious of the apple turnovers, the danish, and the cookies, although I have seen a few varieties of cookies that are milk-free in a special box for kids.

13. I would feel pretty safe with the fries, curly and straight. Likewise, the hash browns, potato cakes, and potato nuggets. But checking for ingredients is not a bad idea.

14. At the new broasted chicken restaurants, there are a variety of choices. Your child should be able to eat the chicken and several of the side dishes, including the pureed squash, baked potato, corn on the cob, coleslaw, applesauce, green beans, three bean salad, fruit salad, clear gelatin salads, and baked beans. Skip the biscuits, dinner rolls, and corn bread.

15. At the ice-cream parlor or in the mall, look for nondairy sorbet. Be sure and ask about sorbet ingredients because some contain cream. Also, many yogurt outlets now carry dairy-free frozen desserts such as This Is Blis or Colombo's Breezer.

16. Remember that soda pop is milk free, and so is orange juice, lemonade, and the red juice that swirls around in many beverage containers. The purple stuff is milk-free also.

Most parents who write to me about fast-food restaurants indicate that after some trial and error, they are generally able to put together a menu for their children at any number of the fast-food restaurants across the country. And once they do that, their children find comfort in knowing that there are fun foods awaiting them at the local drive-through.

The following is a list of some of the large fast-food chains along with their addresses and phone numbers, which you can use to obtain more information. I have also included a list of some of the milk-free food items that are available at those chains, based on information I was able to obtain. If there are no foods listed, that does not mean that there are no acceptable foods at that restaurant. Check with your local restaurant for milk-free options. Also, please be aware that since publication, some of this information may have changed. If you need to be completely vigilant about milk and its components in foods, it is best to check frequently with your local restaurant manager to be sure of the milk content in a variety of food choices.

Milk-Free Fast-Food Choices

A & W International
922 Broadway
Santa Monica, CA 90406

> Hamburger
> Root beer

Baskin Robbins
PO Box 1200
Glendale, CA 91209

> Daiquiri ice
> Grape ice
> Lime ice
> Raspberry sorbet
> Boysenberry sorbet

Burger King Corporation
Consumer Relations Mail Station 1490
PO Box 520783, General Mail Facility
Miami, FL 33152
305-596-7320

> Hamburger buns
> Whopper/Burger patty is 100 percent beef
> B-K Broiler without sauce
> Ham, sausage, and bacon
> Condiments
> Tartar sauce
> Barbecue sauce
> Horseradish sauce
> Sweet and sour sauce
> French fries
> Hash browns
> Thousand island dressing
> Reduced-calorie Italian dressing

Dunkin Donuts
PO Box 317
Randolph, MA 02368

> Most likely, there will be no milk-free offerings here.

Hardees Research and Development Department
1233 Hardee's Blvd.
Rocky Mount, NC 27804-2815
919-977-8506

> Turkey club
> Chef salad without cheese
> French fries
> Apple turnover
> Big cookie
> Fried egg
> Hamburger

Jack in the Box Foods
Foodmaker Inc.
Quality Assurance Department
PO Box 783
San Diego, CA 92112
619-571-2384

> Apple turnover
> Barbecue sauce
> Bacon
> Beef patty
> Breakfast ham
> Canadian-style bacon
> English muffin
> French fries
> Gourm-Egg
> Hamburger buns
> Hamburger seasoning
> Hash browns
> Kaiser roll
> Condiments
> Mushroom topping
> Mayo-onion sauce
> Onion bun
> Pancake syrup
> Pasta salad
> Pita and rye bread
> Shrimp
> Salsa
> Seafood cocktail sauce

continues

Secret sauce
Tartar sauce
Tortilla chips
Tortilla shell and meat filling
Turkey
Vegetable shortening
Wedge fries
Wheat bun
Whitefish and crab blend

Kentucky Fried Chicken
PO Box 32070
Louisville, KY 40323-2070
502-456-8300

Rotisserie chicken
Side dishes such as applesauce, green beans, and corn

McDonald's Corporation
Nutrition Information Center
Oak Brook, IL 60521

Big Mac (without cheese)
Beef patty
Hamburger bun
Condiments
French fries
Big Mac sauce
Barbecue sauce
Bacon
Chef salad (without cheese)
Chicken salad (without cheese)
Shrimp salad (without cheese)
Side salad

Wendy's International Inc.
PO Box 256
4288 W. Dublin Granville Rd.
Dublin, OH 43017
614-764-3100

Hamburger patties
Hamburger buns

Grilled chicken sandwich
Bacon
Condiments
Chili
French fries
Salad bar
Bread sticks
Coleslaw
Celery seed dressing
French dressing
Golden Italian dressing
Thousand Island dressing
Reduced-calorie Italian dressing
Fish fillet
Taco salad (without cheese or sour cream)
Tartar sauce
French toast
Breakfast potatoes
Sausage patties
Syrup
Wheat toast
Liquid margarine

Eating in Restaurants

Children are taken to restaurants every day in this country, and a dairy sensitivity should certainly not stop you from enjoying this experience with your child. Today it seems that everyone is on some kind of a restricted diet, and restaurant chefs, wait staff, and management are all accustomed to special requests and inquiries about ingredients of menu items. There is nothing unusual or rude about asking the restaurant personnel to help you make dairy-free choices for your child. It is important, however, not to guess. Sometimes the wait staff is unsure about specific ingredients in a menu item or will answer your question very tentatively. In that case, simply ask your server to double check with the chef. Unfortunately for some children with severe allergies, there may be hidden ingredients in foods that even the best chef is unaware of.

I recently received a letter from a mother who had taken her lactose-intolerant daughter out for lunch and after checking with the waiter, felt quite comfortable about ordering a tuna-fish sandwich for her. Later that afternoon, the little girl became quite ill with stomach pain and diarrhea. The mother called the restaurant back, spoke with the chef herself, and discovered that, sure enough, sour cream was a standard ingredient in the tuna salad.

I have seen a similar situation happen in the case of a milk-protein-allergic child. Unknown to the parents, some tuna fish contains added milk proteins. If the product is kosher and is manufactured by a major company in the United States, its label will carry a *U* in a circle, followed by a *D* denoting that the product is kosher and contains a milk component. In the case of tuna fish, the milk component is milk protein sometimes added to the fish broth. The parents I am speaking of ordered a tuna-fish sandwich for their child in a restaurant, feeling quite certain that tuna fish surely did not contain milk. Because they could not scrutinize the label, they were unfortunately mistaken. Their daughter had an allergic reaction.

Children whose food allergies cause them to react severely to foods are in particular danger, even when eating at home. Hidden ingredients are in so many manufactured items, even those that are minimally processed, that it is probably impossible to completely protect your child. Instead, your child's pediatric allergist will most likely recommend that the child be given an adrenaline injection kit to be made available at all times in case of an allergic emergency. However, even for these children, these are some strategies for eating in restaurants safely.

1. Before you order, let the wait staff know that your child's meal is not to contain any dairy foods. Spell it out. Be specific. Let them know that you do not want your child to have any milk, cheese, sour cream, or butter.

2. If a dish contains a dairy product, see if that product can be omitted. In other words, see if the restaurant can make your child a taco without the cheese and sour cream. Even pizza can be ordered without cheese.

3. Order the toast or bagel dry; your child can enjoy it with jelly or jam.

4. Order every sandwich and salad without cheese, and ask that all sautéed or grilled fish, meat, or poultry be prepared with oil instead of butter.

5. Choose simple foods for your child: broiled entrées, boiled or baked potato, steamed or sautéed vegetables without any butter. If it's spaghetti your child loves, make sure the marinara sauce is made without cheese.

6. Some desserts are milk-free such as angel food cake, fruit pies, pecan pie, lemon meringue pie, and baked or fresh fruit. Choose from one of those.

7. When selecting a soup, choose a broth-based soup, rather than a cream-based soup. Chicken soup with noodles, matzo balls, rice, or vegetables is great. So is beef soup with vegetables or barley. Lentil and tomato soups are often milk-free, but check to be sure. Any soup (or other dish, for that matter) labeled vegan is completely meat and dairy-free. Veganism is a type of vegetarianism in which no animal products whatsoever are eaten.

8. A variety of salad dressings are milk-free. These include vinaigrette without cheese, oil and vinegar you pour on yourself, oily Italian dressings, Thousand Island, dark red French, and usually orange French, as well. Skip the ranch, creamy garlic, and blue cheese.

Use the following guide to help you make choices in so-called ethnic restaurants:

Cajun   Many cajun dishes are milk-free. However, some of the signature sauces contain cream or milk along with their roux bases. Stick to the simple Cajun dishes such as blackened fish, red beans and rice, gumbo soup, jambalaya, and shrimp creole. Skip all sauces and gravies because they are usually made with milk.

Chinese   Lots of choices here! Chinese cooking is almost completely devoid of all dairy foods. Choose all the stir-fry dishes, chicken-stock-based soups, egg rolls, spring rolls, and fried or boiled wontons. Enrich your child's choice with calcium by selecting a dish that contains tofu—either in soup or in the stir-fry meal. Enjoy lots of great tasting vegetables and fried noodles, which kids love. The sizzling soups and dishes are made from special milk-free noodles. Watch out for the crabmeat rangoons and other seafood specialties in which cream cheese or sour cream is added, such as shrimp toasts. But, for the most part, almost everything on the menu is safe here.

French   There are very few choices here. The chateaubriand is usually a beef fillet, sautéed in butter, but you may be able to ask for it dry or prepared in oil instead. Ratatouille is a vegetable dish that contains eggplant, tomato, onions, and mushrooms, and is often made milk-free. Sometimes, though, it does contain cheese. Beef bourguignonne is a ragout made with beef, mushrooms, onions, and red wine. It may, however, contain cream. The bread sticks should be fine.

Greek   The stuffing in stuffed grape leaves is generally milk-free; it is made from minced meat, spices, and rice. Also a gyro served without yogurt should be fine. A gyro is a sandwich consisting of a processed lamb or beef product served with onion and sauce wrapped in pita bread. Without the sauce, it is milk-free. Also a Greek salad served without cheese is acceptable. The dressing is an oil and vinegar base.

Indian   Foods made from traditional Indian recipes are milk-free and also contain no meat. These vegetarian dishes are highly seasoned with a variety of unusual spices, which many children enjoy.

Italian   There are limited choices here, too. However, you may be able to order pizza without cheese, pasta with a cheese-free marinara sauce, chicken cacciatore without romano cheese, melon proscuitto, Italian bread and bread sticks, which can be dipped in seasoned olive oil, and a green salad. Some children like plain pasta lightly seasoned with oil. It's nutritious, filling, and milk-free.

Japanese   Asian cooking is almost always milk-free. There are many choices here, including grilled meats and vegetables served with rice or noodles. Some children love sushi. It's milk-free and the seaweed is packed with calcium!

Mexican   These restaurants offer many options for dairy-sensitive children because many of the dishes that typically contain cheese and sour cream can be ordered plain. For example, your child can enjoy fajitas, tacos, burritos, and flautas, all prepared without cheese or sour cream. Guacamole is milk-free, as is salsa, picante sauce, taco sauce, tortilla chips, tortillas, chili, and gazpacho. Spanish rice and refried beans are also milk-free.

Middle Eastern   Again, the Middle Eastern diet is basically milk-free with the exception of yogurt, a food used liberally to spoon on top of meats and vegetables. Many Middle Eastern dishes can be enjoyed without the yogurt such as schwarmas, shish-kebab, and dolmas (stuffed grape leaves). Hummus, a wonderfully nutritious and calcium-rich spread made from chickpeas, is milk-free, as is babaganous, a spread made from eggplant. Lentil salad, couscous, tabouli salad, and rice pilaf are all milk-free. Tahini, a spread made from sesame seeds, is calcium-rich as well as milk-free and is wonderful on pita bread or crackers.

Spanish   A variety of dishes made in the Mediterranean Spanish tradition are milk-free, including boiled fish dishes and seafood dishes such as paella, a combination of shrimp, rice, peas, mussels, and other seafoods. Tapas, which is the traditional name for the complement of antipasto-type foods served before the meal are often milk-free. Tapas might include eggplant dip, olives and peppers, seafood in tomato sauce, and lavash bread or crackers. Many other Spanish dishes are made from potatoes, eggs, and chopped tomatoes.

Szechuan This Asian style of cooking is similar to Mandarin or Cantonese Chinese foods, but contains a variety of mildly hot to very hot peppers in the sauces. These foods are also generally milk-free, with very few exceptions.

Thai Another Asian cuisine, Thai food is made up of many types of sautéed or stir-fried meats, seafoods, and poultry combined with vegetables and often peanuts. Generally, Thai food is milk-free.

7

To Market,
to Market

The children's nursery rhyme tells of how, in the very old days, parents went "to market, to market, to buy a fat pig..." Unfortunately, despite admonishments, parents are still going to market and buying fat pigs, fat cows, fat snacks, and fat desserts. This is a real issue today. Dr. Donald M. Black, director of the Preventive Cardiology Clinic in the Division of Pediatric Cardiology at the University of Michigan Medical Center, reports: "It used to be that 80 percent of the kids we were seeing had high cholesterol due to genetics, and the others were due to obesity. Now, it's closer to 50/50." Half the children being seen by pediatric cardiologists today have high cholesterol levels because of genetic components they inherit. But the other half of these children have impaired cardiac function because they are obese—because they exercise too little and eat too much fat.

One of the main obstacles to good cardiac health in children is the school lunch program, according to Patricia J. Goshorn, R.D., clinic dietitian at the University of Michigan. A recent U.S. Department of Agriculture study reported that school lunches contain 25 percent too much fat and 100 percent too much sodium. A significant high fat component in the school lunch program is whole milk—thankfully, something your child will not be consuming. The USDA has developed a plan to improve the nutritional quality of school lunches, but it will not be implemented until 1998. Experts advise that children are better off bringing a healthy lunch from home, if they can. This advice places the responsibility for a child's nutrition squarely on the shoulders of his or her parents, even when the child is in school.

Recently, the *American Journal of Clinical Nutrition* reported the findings of a study that revealed that "Fatty snacks, such as chips and packaged cookies, were reported favorites of obese kids, whereas the non-obese like high carbohydrate snacks, such as popsicles and soft drinks." In other words, leaner kids preferred sugary snacks, as opposed to the fat-laden snacks preferred by the obese children. In comparing the two groups, both the lean children and the obese children ate about the same number of calories. The difference clearly was in the origin of the calories: Children fared better when calories were derived from sugar rather than when calories were derived from fat. I am not advocating feeding children large quantities of sugary snacks, but when children are faced with a choice between sugar and fat, the nonfat solution should be chosen.

Parents need to be aware of this information because it is they who buy the food their children will eat. The current expert recommendations are that after the age of two, when a child's most explosive growth has concluded, parents should monitor their child's fat intake to avoid obesity and elevated blood cholesterol levels, thereby protecting their child's cardiovascular system from components likely to cause damage in adulthood. At the root of this recommendation is food shopping and preparation. Parents need to learn how to make healthy choices in the marketplace and protect those choices by preparing foods without adding lots of fats and oils.

Parents of dairy-sensitive children face another challenge in the marketplace as well. They must look for and avoid milk and its by-products in all processed and packaged foods. This means reading labels, probably thousands of labels over the course of a year. So, this chapter will take parents "to market, to market," but unlike parents of old, who went to "buy a fat pig," you will learn how to choose lean foods as well as dairy-free foods and foods appropriate for meals at home and at school.

Making Healthy Food Choices

Choosing foods for your dairy-sensitive child differs very little from choosing foods for your entire family. Everyone should be eating a variety of meats, fruits, vegetables, breads, and whole grains, and these foods should be as fresh as possible, with as little processing as possible. Foods are best prepared with minimal added salt, sugar, and fat. Foods should be baked or broiled rather than fried, and fatty or sugary snacks and desserts kept to a minimum. Sounds easy, right? Well, it is easy, if you know how to make healthy choices from the unbelievable variety of foods in today's supermarket.

So, come with me to the supermarket and imagine that you are walking alongside my grocery cart. Soon, you will see how easy it is to go from the entrance to the checkout line and end up with a cart chock-full of healthy and milk-free food choices. . . .

Let's admire the first display we see of specialty cakes prepared by the supermarket bakery. So many to choose from! There are decorated cakes, coffee cakes, pies, and muffins. There may even be a "Buy One—Get One Free" promotion going on today. Unless the special is on angel food cake or sponge cake, which are both low in fat and milk-free, we will not buy anything here. Most of these baked goods are made with milk and are not suitable for our family. But wait, there is an angel food cake on the next table. We will buy one to serve with fresh strawberries and dairy-free whipped cream. That will make a nice treat for the kids.

Next we walk into the produce department; we need to spend the most time shopping here, selecting fruits and vegetables, packaging our choices, perhaps weighing our choices. Everything here is milk-free, and we will choose a variety of fresh fruits for snacking and to accompany our meals. Perhaps we'll put together a nice fruit salad made by combining chunks of apples, oranges, and bananas with a bit of mayonnaise, just to make it creamy. Don't forget the strawberries for the angel food cake. The vegetables we choose today include broccoli, as part of dinner tonight, and bok choy, which we will stir-fry with julienne carrots and zucchini later in the week. We also pick out a few ripe avocados, which are rich in so many nutrients. Some people are afraid to serve avocados because they are high in fat, but really, the fat derived from this fruit (yes, it is a fruit!) is almost completely unsaturated (good for the heart!). One avocado contains 630 to 880 IU of healthy vitamin A and 600 mg of potassium, along with more than 1000 µg of pantothenic acid (a very important B vitamin) and 420 µg of Vitamin B_6. We will use the avocados to make guacamole as a topping for the tacos we will cook on Wednesday.

Next we move into the brand-name bread department, where we select an ethnic type, perhaps pita, Italian, or French, as well as a calcium-fortified milk-free white or wheat bread. We'll take an extra one for the freezer. We skip the croissants, the buttered garlic bread, and the sweet rolls. Now we pass the refrigerated lunch meat section. Here, we select low-fat turkey or ham, but skip the bologna, salami, pepperoni, and pork hot dogs. We definitely skip the beef jerky strips and the liverwurst. We might try a low-fat kosher beef hot dog product, which is always milk-free, and makes a nice, quick, lunch that kids or baby-sitters can prepare easily. The kids won't be served hot dogs too frequently, but once in a while should be okay.

As we continue around the aisles, we select condiments such as ketchup, mustard, and mayonnaise. We might prefer a low-fat or light mayonnaise, but don't really worry about it too much because we use so little as it is, preferring instead to spread our children's sandwiches with mustard, barbecue sauce, or hummus, all of which are fat-free and milk-free. Besides, the kids do need some fat for growth. We might pick up some pickles, olives, or relish for the hot dogs we just bought.

In the canned food aisle, we select salmon, sardines, and shrimp, for sure. We will use these canned fish and seafood products to make sandwich spreads, to toss into salads, and to make dips for cut-up vegetables. We might even try to find a recipe for homemade salmon ravioli to prepare over the weekend. We pick up some canned okra to toss in the soup, because there wasn't any fresh today, and some mustard greens to serve as a side dish. Maybe we will make twice-baked potatoes and blend the cooked greens into the potato mixture. It tastes great!

As we pass the ethnic foods such as Mexican, Chinese, and Kosher, we toss a few more things into our cart, such as fat-free, vegetarian refried beans, salsa, chopped mild chiles, and taco seasoning. We will pick up the flour tortillas when we get to the refrigerated section. Soft-shell tacos are a favorite in our house! We also pick up some water chestnuts and bean sprouts for the stir-fry, to go along with the bok choy we already bought in the produce section. From the kosher foods we buy low-fat chicken stock to use as soups or in making sauces; a package of matzo-ball mix or egg noodles for a hearty soup (soup is always a great lunch—and a great way to use leftovers); some beef or chicken bouillon cubes, which are always milk-free if they are kosher; and some kasha, a whole-grain side dish. Also, here we will find a parve chicken coating mix for baking fried chicken. All the items marked kosher-parve are completely milk-free, and there are lots to choose from.

Passing by the meat counter, we pick up a low-fat flank steak for grilling, some cut-up chicken for baking, a combination of one half ground turkey and one half ground sirloin for the taco meat, and a frozen turkey with no added lactose or milk-protein solution for the upcoming holiday. In the fish department, we select whatever is the special of the day, as long as it is not breaded. We needn't linger in the cereal department. Shopping here is quick and easy. We always get some oatmeal, Cream of Wheat, and a couple of dry cereals for snacking. We do not buy the toaster treats because, even though they are next to the breakfast cereal, this product is not an appropriate breakfast food, and they often contain milk. If the kids want a sort of Danish, they can have a piece of toast with milk-free margarine and jelly, or a piece of toast spread with milk-free margarine and sprinkled with a cinnamon and sugar mixture. This is a great snack for midafternoon and is even healthier if we use calcium-enriched bread and serve calcium-enriched apple juice with it.

Down the cookie and cracker aisle, we do get a package of graham crackers and a package of saltines. We won't buy any packaged chocolate-chip cookies, but we can make our own milk-free chocolate-chip cookies this weekend using semisweet chocolate morsels that contain no milk sugar or milk protein. Now that we're thinking about it, maybe we should pick up a package of marshmallows and some milk-free dark chocolate to go along with the graham crackers and make s'mores instead. As we turn the corner, we've entered the chip aisle. We will buy a bag of plain popcorn, pretzels, or baked tortilla chips for snacking. These are all low in fat and many varieties are milk-free. Actually, we might buy all three and let the kids make assorted little packages of these snacks to toss into their lunchboxes for school. Sounds like a fun weekend activity for them, and it saves a lot of work for us.

In the pharmacy aisle, we will pick up some chewable lactase enzyme tablets for our lactose-intolerant teenager, who can digest about two pieces of pizza with the enzyme's help. We will also pick up a flavored, chewable calcium carbonate product like Tums for all of us, from the three-year-old to grandma, to help supplement our calcium intake. We won't worry about the antacid designation on the package. These antacids are strictly calcium carbonate, nothing more, no medicine of any kind. Oh, let's not forget the lactose-free children's chewable vitamins for the three-year-old, who doesn't seem to be eating much of anything worthwhile these days. We try to limit her juice intake and offer her lots of food choices, but she just doesn't seem to be very interested. Oh well, the doctor says she is fine, just going through a finicky stage. Luckily, she does love peanut butter and banana sandwiches. But who knows how long that will last!

Don't make the mistake of passing up the dairy aisle. Here you will find a variety of tofu products, soft tofu for blending with raspberries to make a terrific breakfast food and hard tofu for using in the stir-fry. We will cube the tofu and mix it with a variety of cut-up vegetables to stir-fry in sesame oil and soy sauce. In the dairy case, we also find a dairy-free cheese product, made from casein (suitable for our lactose-intolerant kids, but not for those with a milk-protein allergy). There are also several varieties of Veganrella mock cheese products made from almonds. Or we might select a cheese alternative made from soy products. We'll have to try several different ones before choosing our favorites. We make a note to go to the local whole food store or health food store to check out their selection of alternative cheese products. Don't forget the lactose-reduced milk for those who can drink it.

Now we're rounding the frozen food corner. Here, we pick up some dairy-free frozen treats such as Popsicles, Mocha Mix, and Tofutti. We might want to try the Mama Tish's frozen fruit treats, or the Dole frozen fruit products. The manager of the store, who knows that we're always on the lookout for dairy-free foods, comes over to say hello and tells us that very soon a new product from California called This Is Blis will be in the store. It's a dairy-free soft ice cream product that comes in a variety of flavors. He'll let us know when it arrives.

Also in the frozen food section we find packages of frozen bagels, practically a staple in our home, milk-free frozen bread dough for home-baked flavor, and a variety of kosher-parve soups such as vegetable barley, potato, and cabbage soup. We can also buy some milk-free pie crust, pastry shells, or phyllo dough, terrific for making apple strudel or vegetable strudel. Somehow, everything tastes better when wrapped in phyllo dough, even salmon spread! Also in this section we find milk-free artificial creamers that are useful when added in small quantities as a milk substitute in a variety of cooked or baked dishes. This product easily replaces the evaporated milk in pumpkin pie, and no one can ever tell the difference. We also use it for preparing milk-free butter-cream frosting, but it's not absolutely necessary. Warm water or orange juice works just as well.

As we pass through the checkout counter and make our way to the parking lot with about ten bags of groceries, we are feeling pretty good about our choices and glad that our shopping is finished for the week. It is then we realize that we did not buy the calcium-fortified frozen orange juice or the baby's formula. Darn it! We always forget something! Oh well, we'll just have to come back tomorrow.

The following should help you make healthy choices in the market. Table 7.1 gives you some ideas for exchanging high fat foods for lower fat alternatives. Replacing the fatty choice with the leaner choice does not mean that flavor or satisfaction has to be diminished, as you will easily see.

Table 7.1   Healthy Alternatives to Fatty Foods

INSTEAD OF:	CHOOSE:
Bacon	Canadian bacon, lean ham
Beef hot dog	Chicken or turkey dog
Big Mac	Grilled chicken sandwich
Bran muffin	Bagel, toast, English muffin
Butter/margarine/cream cheese	Jam, jelly, preserves, apple or other fruit butters
Cake/pie/cookies/pastries	Angel food, sponge cake, baked apple, fruit crisp, oatmeal cookies, ginger snaps, fruit (fresh or juice packed)
Chili con carne	Chili made from ground turkey
Chocolate candy	Chocolate sauce on fruit or sponge cake
Coleslaw	Shredded cabbage with vinaigrette
Cookies	Fig bars, flavored rice cakes
Corned beef/pastrami	Smoked turkey, turkey ham
Croissant	Bagel, toast, English muffin
Doughnut	Angel food cake, cinnamon toast, toast with jelly or jam
Egg noodles	Macaroni, plain pasta
French fries	Baked or roasted potatoes
Fried foods	Baked, broiled, steamed, or roasted meat, fish, poultry, and vegetables
Ice cream/frozen yogurt	Milk-free sorbet
Oils/salad dressings	Mustard, ketchup, barbecue sauce

INSTEAD OF:	CHOOSE:
Oil-packed tuna	Water-packed tuna
Mayonnaise	Reduced-calorie salad dressings, hummus spread for sandwiches
Lamb chop	Leg of lamb
Potato chips	Pretzels, rice cakes, melba toast, air-popped or microwave popcorn
Pork spare ribs	Pork loin
Roast duck	Roast chicken
Roasted peanuts	Chestnuts
Sour cream on tacos	Salsa

Fat in All Its Forms

When reading labels, use this information to guide you in the selection of appropriate and healthy choices for your child. Remember that growing children need some fat in their diet for a variety of physiological processes and to meet their high energy needs. The following list should help you choose more healthful fats such as monounsaturated fats or polyunsaturated fats rather than saturated fats or hydrogenated fats. In general, fats derived from plant sources such as vegetables and soy are healthful fats, while fats derived from meat or dairy sources are definitely not as desirable.

Cholesterol A chemical compound manufactured in the body used to build cell membranes and brain and nerve tissues. Helps the body make steroid hormones and bile acids.

Dietary cholesterol Cholesterol found in animal products such as egg yolks, liver, meat, some shellfish, and dairy products.

Fatty acid   These are the building blocks of fats, composed of carbon and hydrogen atoms.

Fat   One or more fatty acids combine to form a fat. Fat is one of the three main constituents of food along with protein and carbohydrate. It is the principal form in which energy is stored in the body.

Hydrogenated fat   A fat that has undergone a chemical change due to the addition of hydrogen atoms. Vegetable oil and margarine are examples of hydrogenated fat.

Lipid   Chemical compounds insoluble in water including both fat and cholesterol. Other members of the lipid group include fatty acid and phospholipids.

Lipoprotein   A chemical combination of protein and fat. Low-density lipoproteins (LDLs) have more fat than protein, and high-density liproproteins (HDLs) have more protein than fat. These compounds are found in the blood and their main function is to carry cholesterol.

Monounsaturated fatty acid   Found mostly in plant and seafoods, these are fatty acids missing one pair of hydrogen atoms.

Monounsaturated fat   Fats made from monounsaturated fatty acids such as olive oil and canola oil. These fats tend to lower LDL cholesterol levels in the blood.

Polyunsaturated fatty acid   Found mostly in plant and seafoods, these are fatty acid missing more than one pair of hydrogen atoms.

Polyunsaturated fat   Fats made from polyunsaturated fatty acids such as safflower oil and corn oil. These fats tend to lower levels of both HDL cholesterol and LDL cholesterol in the blood.

Saturated fatty acid   Fatty acid which is saturated with hydrogen atoms. This fatty acid has the maximum possible number of hydrogen atoms attached to every carbon atom. It is found in meat and many dairy products.

Saturated fat   Butter and lard are examples of fats that are made from saturated fatty acids. Saturated fats are found in all meat and dairy products, unless the product is fat-free. These fats raise the level of LDL cholesterol in the blood. Elevated levels of LDL are associated with heart disease.

Trans fatty acid   These are polyunsaturated fatty acids in which some of the missing hydrogen atoms have been put back through a chemical process called hydrogenation. They are found mostly in margarine and vegetable oil products. Trans fatty acids are the building blocks of hydrogenated fats.

Reading Food Labels

Getting all the information you need out of a food label isn't always possible. First of all, some foods are not required to carry labels. Currently, only about 60 percent of the products now carried in our markets are required to have a food label. Nutrition information is voluntary for many raw foods, including fresh fruits, vegetables, and fish. Under the Nutrition Labeling and Education Act of 1990 (NLEA), the following foods are exempt from nutrition labeling:

- Foods produced by very small businesses
- Restaurant food
- Food served for immediate consumption, such as that served in hospital cafeterias and airplanes
- Ready-to-eat food prepared primarily on-site such as bakery, deli, and candy-store items
- Food sold by food-service vendors such as mall cookie counters, sidewalk vendors, and vending machines

- Food shipped in bulk, as long as it is not for sale in that form to consumers
- Medical foods, such as those used to address the nutritional needs of patients with certain diseases
- Plain coffee and tea, some spices, and other foods that contain no significant amounts of any nutrients
- Packages with less than twelve square inches available for labeling, although an address or telephone number must be printed for consumers to obtain nutrition information
- Game meat nutritional information may be provided on counter signs, placards, or other point-of-purchase materials

Given these exceptions, it is impossible for you to have complete nutritional or ingredient information about all of the foods your child will likely be eating. You must be prepared, then, to encounter surprise episodes of allergic reactions or digestive distress from your children who are either allergic to milk protein or are lactose intolerant. You will not always know for certain whether milk or a milk by-product is a constituent in your child's food by simply studying the label. The same is true for other allergies as well, such as corn, tomato, soy, or peanuts. As long as your child is eating food, whether it comes from a market or is being served in a restaurant, there is always a possibility that he or she will consume something offensive.

At times, you will have to play detective, speaking with the food-service director, or speaking with the chef, or calling the manufacturer for more complete information. Even so, many products are made from mixes that may contain milk proteins or lactose. The ingredients in these mixes may even be unknown to the food manufacturer, unless a specific ingredient search has been conducted. For example, a common, basic dough mix used by your local bakery might include whey, although no additional milk is added to the baked product. The owner of the bakery might assure you that no milk is in the bread, because none was added, but he or she may be unaware that the dairy by-product whey is a constituent of the commercially prepared mix. If you need to know for certain, you can obtain the name and number of the company that produces the dough mix and get a list of the ingredients. It's work, but finding a nondairy commercial product offers an alternative to baking your own bread from scratch. For the most part, companies are happy to work with consumers, but occasionally you might encounter a difficult manufacturer or an ingredient list that is hard to pin down.

When you are in the supermarket, however, you will mostly encounter foods that offer a federally approved food label. Current food labeling standards refer to both the principal display panel (PDP), which is the part of the label consumers see first when they purchase a product, and the information panel, which is usually to the immediate right of the PDP. Two recent laws have become effective that determine the information required to be printed on the PDP and the information panel. The American Technology Preeminence Act of 1991 requires food manufacturers to list the net contents of their products in both metric units and traditional measurements such as inches and pounds. The Nutrition Labeling and Education Act of 1990 (NLEA) requires nutrition information on almost all foods, a new format for presenting that nutrition information, definitions for nutrient claims such as low-fat, appropriate use of health claims, and ingredient listing on all foods with two or more ingredients. These regulations, which represent the most extensive changes in food labeling history, are designed to make label information more complete and useful than ever before. But they do not make the labels perfect, especially for people looking for lactose or allergens.

The information panel is made up of four parts. First, you will see the Nutrition Facts, which must include:

- Serving size
- Servings per container
- Total calories per serving

- Calories derived from fat per serving
- Total fat amount per serving
- Saturated fat amount per serving
- Cholesterol amount per serving
- Sodium amount per serving
- Total carbohydrate per serving
- Dietary fiber per serving
- Sugars per serving
- Protein per serving
- Vitamin A per serving
- Vitamin C per serving
- Calcium per serving
- Iron per serving

The Nutrition Facts also list the total fat, saturated fat, cholesterol, sodium, carbohydrate, fiber, vitamin A and C, calcium and iron as percentages, representing the percentage of the recommended daily allowance of these nutrients for a 2,000 to 2,500 calorie-per-day diet. You will have to judge for yourself how relevant this information is for your child. The age of your child, whether he is three or thirteen, will determine the approximate number of calories he will be taking in and where these recommended daily allowances fit. Certainly, although it looks quite scientific, these percentage measurements are only meant as guidelines. Will some of this information merely confuse you? Perhaps. But will this information be useful to you? Most definitely. If nothing else, you will be able to use the Nutrition Facts guide to help assess a food for its vitamin and mineral content as well as for its saturated fat content. If you are looking for calcium, the food label will point it out to you. If you are looking for healthy fats or fiber or iron, the food label will help you locate the products you need.

In addition to the required nutrient information, the following information may be included by food manufacturers on a voluntary basis:

- Calories from saturated fat
- Polyunsaturated fat per serving
- Monounsaturated fat per serving
- Potassium per serving
- Soluble fiber per serving
- Insoluble fiber per serving
- Sugar alcohol (xylitol, mannitol, sorbitol) per serving
- Other carbohydrate per serving
- Other essential vitamins and minerals per serving

Part of the goal of the new food labeling requirements is also to encourage food manufacturers to product healthier foods. Posting all of the undesirable ingredients in each package right on the label for all to see gives incentive for change. Potentially food manufacturers will be competing against each other to produce the healthiest form of their product, and in fact, we have seen this happen in the marketplace already.

The other three required sections of the information panel are the company name and address, the copyright symbol, and the ingredient listing. Undoubtedly, the ingredient information is perhaps the most important information for parents of dairy-sensitive children.

Ingredient Listing

The government requires what it terms "full ingredient labeling on standardized foods." This refers to all foods that have more than one ingredient. The ingredient label must also include FDA-certified color additives by name, where appropriate. The label must include sources of protein hydrolysates, which are used in many foods as flavors and flavor enhancers. With respect to milk protein, the government requires that if caseinate is used in a food claiming to be nondairy, the label must declare caseinate to be a "milk derivative."

The entire issue of nondairy labeling is interesting in and of itself. Legally, products may be declared nondairy if they contain no recognizable dairy foods, such as cream or milk. Therefore, many nondairy foods, such as nondairy sour cream, nondairy creamer, and nondairy whipped topping, are often confused with milk-free foods, which they clearly are not because they contain milk by-products offensive to children and adults who are either lactose intolerant or allergic to milk protein. In addition, current regulations do not require manufacturers to inform the public about many milk by-products with the exception of caseinate. For example, whey, as you know, contains both lactose and milk protein, yet it is a constituent of many, many nondairy foods. But whey is not required to carry an explanatory "milk-derivative" statement.

Beatrice Trum Hunter, writing for *Consumer's Research Magazine,* recently explained in an article entitled "The Importance of Ingredient Labeling" how medical cases have been reported of severe milk allergy reactions to several nondairy foods, including frozen tofu, beef hot dogs, bologna, tuna fish, and hypoallergenic infant feeding formulas. She writes that "Investigation showed that in all cases, the offending products contained undeclared casein or caseinate." During the formulation of the new labeling regulations, the government's response to public outcry about this issue was the "caseinate explanatory declaration."

But this does not solve our problem completely, especially for those parents with lactose-intolerant children. Currently, lactose may be part of a sugar component in a particular food, but the government does not require the word "lactose" to appear in the ingredient listing. However, we are seeing more and more manufacturers voluntarily listing the sugar derivative on the label, for example, listing "sugar, derived from dextrose" or "sugar, derived from sucrose." When in doubt, parents may always call the manufacturer for complete information.

Nutrition or Health Claims

There are also new regulations that govern the definitions for terms such as "light" or "low-fat" or "high-fiber" to describe a food's nutritional content. Basically, foods are labled with these descriptive phrases only if they meet the government's uniform standard. Eleven terms have been defined that relate to several nutrients. They are "free," "low," "reduced," "fewer," "lean," "high," "less," "more," "extra lean," "good source," and "light." The term "sodium-free," for example, means that the food contains less than 5 mg of sodium per serving.

Something important to remember is that, currently, the FDA allows "insignificant" amounts of lactose to be present in foods labeled "lactose-free." Whether or not this will change in the future is unknown. The only exception to this rule of standards is 2-percent milk, which can be labeled as

---

Remember That the Following Items Are Derived from Milk:

Calcium caseinate (a milk protein)

Casein (a milk protein)

Lactalbumin (a milk protein)

Lactoglobulin (a milk protein)

Lactose (milk sugar)

Sodium caseinate (a milk protein)

Whey (contains both lactose and milk protein)

Refer to Chapter 2 for tables listing ingredients found on food labels that may or may not be milk by-products.

"low-fat," although it does not meet the government's requirements for low-fat foods. This controversy, which is fast becoming more public, exemplifies the enormous power that dairy industry lobby groups have over legislation that exempts their industry from the rules that apply to all other food manufacturers.

Now for the first time, health claims regarding seven relationships between a nutrient or a food and the risk of a disease or health-related condition will be allowed. These claims may be made based on endorsements from a recognized third-party health reference, such as the National Cancer Institute, or may be made based on the use of statements or symbols, such as a picture of a heart to denote a food approved by the American Heart Association. These health claims may not state the degree of risk reduction and can only use the words "may" or "might" in discussing the nutrient or food and disease relationship. The claims must be clearly phrased so that the average consumer understands the food's relationship to the disease.

Currently, claims may be made for the following food/disease or nutrient/disease relationships:

- Calcium and osteoporosis
- Fat and cancer
- Saturated fat and cholesterol and coronary heart disease
- Fiber-containing grain products, fruits, and vegetables and cancer
- Fruits, vegetables, and grain products that contain fiber and risk of coronary heart disease
- Sodium and high blood pressure
- Fruits and vegetables and cancer

More Helpful Information on the Label

Standard serving sizes   The new food label nutrition information is based on more realistic and standardized serving sizes as well. Through consumer surveys conducted by the government, typical portions were determined for various foods. Therefore you won't find one cookie manufacturer calling a serving size one cookie and another cookie manufacturer calling a serving size two cookies. Like foods are measured according to like serving portions.

Fruit juice amounts Information regarding percentage of actual fruit juice in juice drinks is also now required. Now, when you look at the label of your child's favorite fruit drink, you will know how much of it is actually fruit juice and how much of it is actually colored sugar water.

Grades and standards Some foods, such as eggs, orange juice, and meat, carry a grade on their label that attests to their quality. For eggs, the grades are AA, A, and B. For meats, the words used are "choice" or "select." For more specific information about the quality of foods you want to buy, consult your grocer or butcher for help.

Religious symbols Currently, there are more than fifty symbols that may appear on foods to indicate that the food has been processed according to Jewish dietary laws. Kosher foods must be inspected by a rabbi trained in this type of food preparation, which involves strict cleaning and the complete separation of meat and milk. The difference in symbols is due to the variety of religious organizations that oversee kosher food preparation. But, as discussed earlier, one of the most common symbols is the letter *U* in a circle, which means the food is kosher. If the letter *U* is followed by the letter *D*, that means there is either a dairy component in the food (either lactose or protein or milk fat) or the food was prepared with equipment used in the preparation of milk products. The FDA does not regulate any of these symbols.

Other common symbols on kosher foods are the capital letter *K* in a triangle, or the word "parve." The designation *K* means that the food is kosher. The word "parve" means that the food is parve and may be eaten with either a meat or dairy meal. Because Jewish dietary laws forbid the mixing of meat and dairy within the same meal, all foods labeled parve are milk-free.

Rabbi Yaakov Luban, writing in *Jewish Living* magazine, Summer 1992, brings up a couple of issues about the label designations that may be meaningful for parents of dairy-sensitive children. He informs readers that there may be caseinate present in vegetable broth, typically the type used in canned tuna, and there may also be caseinate in hydrolyzed vegetable protein, often used in soups and seasonings. Also, because current government regulations allow the use of certain general terms, such as "sugar" or "natural flavors" or "artificial flavors," without itemizing each component, trace elements of caseinate or lactose may be present in products listing ingredients in general terms. As you can see, the food labeling system isn't perfect in this country, and parents will just have to do the best they can when trying to eliminate these milk derivatives from their children's food. When in doubt, cook at home and stick to the basics.

Enforcing Label Laws

The FDA, under the leadership of Dr. David Kessler, Commissioner of Food and Drugs, has made a commitment to enforcing these new labeling laws, although the enormity of the task is staggering. However, as recently as last spring, it was reported in the April 20, 1994, issue of the Cleveland *Plain Dealer* that the Keebler Company was recalling a shipment of Ripplin's Original Flavor Potato Snack Chips because an ingredient was not listed on the label. Although the article did not state which specific ingredient was left off the label, it did report that "the chips, marked with the sell-by date of June 28, 1994, may contain milk products not shown in the ingredient statement." Keebler management responded to media inquiry by expressing concern for the risk of allergic reaction among consumers sensitive to milk products, although no illnesses were reportedly linked to the ingestion of the chips. It is probably safe to assume that the milk protein caseinate was the missing ingredient. Grocers withdrew the products from the shelves, and consumers were asked to return the product to the place of purchase for replacement or refund. One month earlier, Keebler recalled its Fudge Shoppe Fudge 'n' Caramel Cookies as a precaution because some may have contained peanut products not listed on the label.

In a study reported in the *Annals of Allergy*, March 1992, a severe allergic reaction occurred in a milk-allergic child after he ate a dairy-free dessert labeled kosher-parve. The two-year-old experienced multiple generalized reactions including elevated levels of milk-specific IgE antibodies in his blood and a strongly positive milk skin test. Working to test the hypothesis that the sorbet he ate contained milk products, although according to the label it should have been milk-free, the scientists determined the milk allergen level in the sorbet to be 11 percent of the level found in nonfat dry milk. The milk allergen level in three independently purchased containers of sorbet ranged from 2 percent to undetectable. The presence of milk in three out of four of the sorbets was confirmed by several laboratory tests. Subsequently, the scientists discovered that milk was incorporated into the sorbet when equipment used to package ice cream had been used to package the sorbet. This incident highlights the importance of vigilant auditing of the food-manufacturing process.

Dr. James E. Gern, of Johns Hopkins University in Baltimore, conducted a study in 1991 that also identified milk proteins in a variety of foods labeled nondairy, including frozen desserts, tuna fish, bologna, and hot dogs. These foods provoked allergic reactions in six children who were otherwise fed strictly milk-free diets. The children reacted with hives, diarrhea, vomiting, and breathing difficulties. Again, milk proteins were the culprits, although their presence in the products was not reflected on the product labels. I believe that this kind of scientific research, which proved so valuable to the ultimate changes required on food labels in this country in 1994, especially with respect to milk protein, was generated from a consumer-based interest in the proper and safe feeding of allergic children. Parents like you can make a difference. For more information about food labeling, or to express your opinions about food labels, you may call or write the following sources:

> Reprints of the Federal Register document containing the regulations are available for $4.50 a set from the United States Government Printing Office at the following address:

GPO—Superintendent of Documents
Washington, DC 20401
202-783-3238

FDA *Consumer Magazine* reports court actions, including seizures and criminal actions, and investigators' reports. It is published by:

Food and Drug Administration
5600 Fishers Lane
Rockville, MD 20857

Milk Coatings on Fruit? A Future Possibility

Because consumers have expressed concern about chemicals in their food, manufacturers are now searching for new ways to preserve food without sacrificing the health of the consumer. While this sounds like a lofty charge, for dairy-sensitive children, these new efforts could prove disastrous. The Agricultural Research Service of the United States Department of Agriculture has been investigating the possibility of making edible coatings from milk and other farm products to keep cut fruits and vegetables fresher longer. It appears that milk protein derived from casein is considered the prime ingredient of such edible coatings. Other foods under investigation for this application include protein derived from soybean, corn, or wheat. If these ingredients are used to make "natural" preservatives, it will surely cause difficulties for parents of children with allergies.

Furthermore, there is no positive assurance that some chemicals won't also be added to the new food coatings. Dominic Wong, of the USDA Western Regional Research Center in Albany, California, explains that "testing is now taking place for an edible food coating made from casein, an emulsifier, and a carbohydrate derived from algae." According to Wong, "it will be a long time before this product will be part of the food marketplace." Still, there is reason for concern. The good intentions of our government may translate into future problems for dairy-sensitive consumers, especially children, whose reactions to milk, soy, corn, or wheat proteins may be severe.

The Subtropical Products Research Laboratory in Florida is considering edible coatings for whole fruits and vegetables that are derived from oils or waxes and cellulose. Currently, some coatings are made from starch, or water-soluble alginate/calcium, carrageenan, and other seaweeds. These coatings may contain potato or tapioca starch, flavorings, or colorings—some of which may be artificial. These coatings are now being used on precooked frozen meat, poultry, and fish. Candies and nuts may be coated with corn protein, vegetable oils, glycerin, and antioxidants, some of which are considered marginally unsafe. All of this information is enough to make even the most relaxed parents frustrated and anxious about shopping for and feeding their children.

Warning: Artificial Sweeteners on the Label

Some parents are vigilant shoppers and do their very best to ensure that their children receive little or no artificial ingredients of any kind in their diet. They shop in whole-food stores and purchase only organically grown fruits, vegetables, and meats with no preservatives present. Other parents are more casual about the use of artificial sweeteners, preferring that their children consume as little sugar as possible, and therefore offering "sugarless" treats such as chewing gum or candy. My position is not to place a value judgment on either of these lifestyles. I personally would opt for feeding children as naturally as possible, but I also understand that it is virtually impossible to keep all of the so-called offensive ingredients out of their lives, especially if children need to take liquid or chewable medications, which are usually artificially sweetened, or will be eating in places other than home. So, if we can presume that your child will be consuming artificial sweeteners, either through food or medicine, you should be aware that some of them may make your child sick with stomach upset. Knowing this ahead of time will help you discern the possible source of your child's diarrhea.

Aspartame   Aspartame was discovered in 1965 and was introduced in the United States as a low-calorie sweetener in 1981. It is found in thousands of products on the market including NutraSweet and Equal. (Prior to 1981, Equal was lactose!) Aspartame is made of two amino acids and methanol, ingredients that occur naturally in some foods, although not in this form. In other words, the components of aspartame are derived from naturally occurring ingredients, but the combination of the three ingredients is not naturally occurring. Aspartame is not suitable for cooking or baking, and is not recommended for individuals with phenylketonuria (PKU), a condition detected at birth. Aspartame has been accused of causing headaches along with a variety of other maladies, including stomach upset. However, a number of scientific studies have been unable to prove a link. In 1984, the Center for Disease Control in Atlanta released statements that cleared the product of any cause-and-effect relationship to these conditions, although there is still some controversy surrounding the product.

Saccharin Saccharin was discovered in 1879 and is a white crystalline powder that is several hundred times sweeter than sugar. It has no caloric content because it passes through the body intact. While saccharin has had a politically checkered history, it is still a very popular sweetener in the United States, although in 1979 it was banned in the manufacture of drugs in Canada. A long history of use has shown that saccharin, consumed in normal amounts, does not have any short-term adverse health effects in humans, except for allergic reactions. However, it has been shown to be a possible cause of bladder cancer in rats. Saccharin is the main ingredient in Sweet 'n Low and has not been identified as causing gastrointestinal symptoms.

Sorbitol Sorbitol is an alcohol derivative of glucose. It occurrs naturally in some berries and fruit, including plums, cherries, and pears. Sorbitol is formed in mammals from glucose and is then converted to fructose. Sorbital is used commercially to sweeten and also to maintain moisture and inhibit crystal formation in some foods. It is also an ingredient in many pharmaceuticals, including pills and liquid medications, and is sometimes used intravenously as a diuretic. It is also found in other sweetened products, such as toothpaste and chewing gum. Commercially, sorbitol is obtained from corn syrup and is therefore not appropriate for people with a corn allergy or a fructose intolerance. It has little effect on the blood sugar level because its rate of absorption is so slow. That's why it may be used by diabetics. However, if taken in excess, it undergoes bacterial fermentation in the large intestine and can produce diarrhea. Sorbitol is not noncaloric, either. It provides about four calories per gram.

Mannitol Mannitol is also a sugar alcohol formed from the reduction of the sugar mannose. Mannitol is present in some plants and fungi and serves a number of pharmaceutical functions, including that of an intravenous diuretic. Commercially, mannitol is frequently present in sugarless chewing gum. It is often paired with sorbitol to sweeten other sugarless foods and candies. Mannitol is poorly absorbed. About 93 percent remains in the intestine, producing an osmotic effect—that is, it draws water, causing diarrhea. The effect is worse when large amounts of mannitol are ingested.

Preserving the Nutrients in Foods

Now that you have worked so hard to shop right and have learned how to select healthy, milk-free choices for your child in the supermarket, the last thing you will want to do is sabotage your good work by preparing foods in a way that destroys nutrients. Here are a few suggestions for getting the most nutrition out of the foods you buy:

1. Vegetables such as broccoli, turnip greens, chard, and salad greens need to be refrigerated in the vegetable crisper or in moisture-proof bags. Their nutrients are best preserved at near-freezing temperatures and at high humidity.

2. Cabbage, a more stable source of vitamin C than most leafy vegetables, should not be allowed to dry out. It should be wrapped or put in the vegetable crisper of the refrigerator where the humidity is high.

3. Tomatoes do best if they are covered with a cloth and ripened out of the sun at room temperature. When they are ripe and firm, they may be kept in the refrigerator for a few days without losing too much of their vitamin C. When the tomatoes are overripe, much of their vitamin content is lost.

4. Fresh green peas and lima beans hold their nutrients best if left in their pods until ready to use. If they are shelled, they should be put into plastic bags and stored in the refrigerator.

5. Carrots, sweet potatoes, potatoes, and other root vegetables and tubers retain their most important nutrients reasonably well if they are kept cool and moist enough to prevent wilting.

6. Freshly dug potatoes contain more vitamin C than stored potatoes. If stored for four months, potatoes can lose up to 60 percent of their vitamin C.

7. Frozen foods are not only equal to fresh foods in nutritional value, but sometimes frozen fruits and vegetables may contain *more* nutrients than fresh. That's because vitamins have a natural tendency to deteriorate when exposed to light or heat. That means every minute between the field and you reduces the nutrients held in the fresh produce. But frozen fruits and vegetables are usually frozen and packaged within four to six hours of being picked. Prior to being frozen, they are "blanched" which means they are tossed into boiling water or steam or hot air for about one to three minutes. This process halts the deterioration of nutrients and preserves the color and flavor of the fresh produce. According to the National Frozen Food Association, fresh green beans retained only 36 percent of their vitamin C content after three days in the display case and three days in the refrigerator at home. This compares to frozen green beans which retained 77 percent of their vitamin C content.

8. Some produce farmers use containers called hydrocoolers that bring the temperature down to the thirties as soon as possible in order to prevent nutrient loss from the field. Check with your grocer to see if their suppliers use this type of equipment.

9. Avoid trimming and cutting fruits and vegetables into small pieces as much as possible. This exacerbates nutrient loss.

10. Avoid cooking vegetables in large amounts of water, which causes the nutrients to leech out. Instead, prepare vegetables in the microwave oven, in a steamer, or as a quick stir-fry.

11. Eat fruits fresh from the refrigerator without cooking.

12. Save the water used to cook vegetables and use it to make mashed potatoes or add to soups and stews. Toss into tomato juice to enrich it.

Suggestions for Getting Your Child to Eat Vegetables

Parents often complain that their children don't eat enough vegetables. In fact, it's true. A study done at Cornell University asked 1,800 second and fifth graders to name everything they had eaten during one twenty-four-hour period. More than half had diets the researchers graded as fair or poor. Half the children failed to meet their recommended daily allowances. Twenty percent ate no fruit at all. Fifteen percent did not eat vegetables and 40 percent liked potatoes only if they were fried, and tomatoes only if they were served in a sauce. Seven percent of the second graders and 16 percent of the fifth graders ate no breakfast at all. Many of the children skipped meals.

It should be noted, however, that in many studies, children of this age often did not consume adequate diets during a twenty-four-hour period, but did somewhat better when their dietary intake was measured over several days. Still, most children could use a little help when it comes to eating their vegetables.

1. Take your child shopping with you. Having your child help you choose foods often piques his or her interest.

2. Grow your own. Eating vegetables is never more fun than when they are grown and picked and eaten straight from your garden. They are also the most nutritious when they are eaten soon after harvesting. If you have never eaten corn or tomatoes or eggplant from your own garden, you are missing something special. Your children will respond positively to your enthusiasm as well.

3. Set a good example. Eat lots of vegetables yourself.

4. Get the kids involved in food preparation. They are more likely to eat something they have had a hand in cooking or chopping or setting out on a plate. Kids can tear lettuce for salad or shell peas or add ingredients to the bowl. They can wash vegetables and place them in the dish for the microwave.

5. Don't serve mush. Crispy, colorful vegetables usually have more appeal. Cook the vegetables, but leave them firm and intact.

6. Serve raw vegetables with a dip as the meal's first course or as a snack.

7. Introduce only one new food at a time. If you want your child to try beets, for example, serve a meal composed of other foods he normally eats, and make the introduction of beets sound a little bit special.

8. Invite your child to try very small portions of new foods, but don't coerce him. You might say, "You can try this if you want to."

9. Think of fun ways to serve vegetables. Cookie cutters can be used to make fun shapes when pressed into slices of cooked squash or raw zucchini.

10. Let your child name the vegetables. For example, he might like to call broccoli "trees" or cauliflower "clouds."

11. Don't assume for one minute that because he didn't like peas on Tuesday, he won't eat peas on Friday. Keep trying. Don't turn his dislike of a vegetable into a long-lasting self-fulfilling prophecy. Give him a chance to grow and change. It may take him three more years to eat peas, but chances are he will . . . someday.

12. If your child is especially finicky, serve fruit. Many fruits provide terrific nutrients for your child, and if they are more easily taken, should be offered several times a day.

13. If all else fails, give your child a vitamin supplement. *Do not* turn mealtime into a war or into some weird psychological exercise. The food on the table is not love or power or respect. It is *food,* to be eaten and enjoyed for the wonderful energy and satisfaction it gives us.

Magic Potions in the Pharmacy

Merlin was a famous magician and prophet, so powerful he was even capable of changing behavior and outcomes. He could make wrong things right again. Today, although our lifestyle is very different from that in King Arthur's court, we continue to attribute many magical qualities to medicine and the people who administer that medicine to us. We often say that medications are "miracle drugs" or "wonder drugs" because the good they can do in so many instances is truly magical. The intelligence and curiosity and perseverance necessary to develop little pills to cure our ills is remarkable. Think of it . . . from plants or fungi or some technological simulation of plant processes or chemical interactions, pharmacists and physicians, chemists and biologists, and other scientists invent medicines that take away our hives, our cramps, and our headaches. Merlin would be proud. Medicine is indeed a magical world, beyond the scope of most people, yet a world that affects each and every adult and child, and a world you as parents of dairy-sensitive infants and children will have to enter.

Generally children in this country enjoy good health. I once had a friend who was a pediatrician. After several years of practice, he went back to medical school to do a residency in dermatology. Why? Because he felt little challenge from his pediatric practice. "Kids," he said, "are basically healthy, and if they do get sick, they usually bounce back pretty quickly." He was looking for more interesting diseases to fight than runny noses and the occasional strep throat. He also did not consider frequent colicky symptoms children often have or hives or fidgetyness a component of disease—at least not diseases he was interested in. Many of you might find his attitude a bit offensive, but the truth is, most children in this country are pretty healthy, although most will likely, at one time or another, have an illness that requires medication. Perhaps your child has already been ill several times in his or her life. Possibly, if your child has experienced several weeks or months of undiagnosed food allergies or intolerances, you have learned quite a bit about medication and medical procedures. Perhaps some aspects of your child's treatment were even a little difficult to endure. Most people give in to the idea that being ill is a part of life, but that doesn't make it any easier for parents coping with a sick child. Besides, some experts disagree completely with this notion.

Dr. Lendon Smith, a prominent pediatrician and author of numerous books about children's medical problems and their relationships to food, has written several best sellers. He has been called America's most trusted pediatrician. One of his books, *Foods for Healthy Kids,* espouses his theory that a child's health is determined by many factors, including the mother's pregnancy, delivery, genetics, nutrition, and environmental stresses. He is a positive believer in the idea that nutrition plays an essential prophylactic role in a child's health; in other words, excellent nutrition will actually prevent illness. Parents need not accept the fact that many diseases are a part of life and should not resign themselves to their children's unwell experiences. Among his patients and their families, many do consider his work to be magical. Dr. Smith and other pediatricians like him may just be a little like Merlin because they treat the whole child and often make wrong things right again. Pediatricians who treat children with a combination of medicine, nutrition therapies, and supportive advice for parents are working the hardest to affect the excellent long-term health of children by paying attention to all the factors that contribute to a child's growth.

Dr. Smith writes, "In my pediatric practice I see many children who simply 'don't feel good.' When they don't feel well, they are likely to become surly, demanding, hyperactive, or withdrawn." He goes on to explain that "Once symptoms appear, we know the child is no longer able to screen out the debilitating stimuli. When the neocortex of the brain senses danger, it signals the pituitary, the adrenals, other organs, and the muscles to help handle the problem. If these organs are overstimulated and not replenished with rest and *adequate nutrition,* illness is the result."

Smith ponders the entire field of medicine, calling it a "very neat and tidy system." But, as a holistic pediatrician, he is concerned not only with diagnosing an illness and prescribing a medicine, but also with trying to figure out what caused the illness in the first place. In the process, he often discovers poorly nourished children. Smith, who is extremely jovial and charming, nevertheless gives serious attention to children who display all kinds of behaviors that may be the result of food allergies and intolerances. He does not dismiss the antics of children who often suck their fingers or rock or are ticklish beyond reason or who have frequent stomachaches or headaches, but rather he gives credence to the presence of these behaviors as symptoms of underlying problems with nourishment.

In April 1995, a most astonishing scientific study was published that offers the very first *clinical proof* that nutrition actually has a physiological affect on disease. Researchers at the University of North Carolina at Chapel Hill and the U.S. Department of Agriculture found that a virus severely damaged the hearts of mice with deficiencies in the mineral selenium, but had no effect on mice that had enough selenium in their diets. According to Dr. Melinda Beck, who directed the research, "It's direct evidence. We saw the virus itself had changed because it was replicated in a selenium-deficient animal." Beck, a viral immunologist and pediatrician at the UNC-CH School of Medicine, worked with Qing Shi of UNC and Dr. Orville Levander and Virginia Morris of the USDA. Beck has asserted that if the findings apply to other viruses, the hypothesis may be tested to explain the evolution of more deadly forms of diseases such as influenza and hepatitis. This study confirms the link between nutrition and viral mutation and shows its molecular basis.

What does this mean to you? Clearly, the responsibility for your child's nutrition lies in your hands; therefore so do some aspects of your child's medical health. Being aware of medical and nutritional information will help you make better decisions and will help support the kind of healthy lifestyle you will ultimately fashion for your child. Being informed, by reading books such as those written by Dr. Lendon Smith, Dr. Doris Rapp, Dr. Benjamin Spock, Dr. Penelope Leach, Dr. T. Berry Brazelton, and other noted pediatricians, and following the health news in journals, magazines, and newspapers will make you better at the job of nurturing and at parenting. One of my pet peeves is people who say, "Well, all parents just do the best they can." But do they really? Do all parents make the same effort?

A very likable woman who I knew in Iowa was referred to me for counseling by her son's pediatrician. I will call her Carol. Carol's baby was diagnosed with a milk-protein allergy at about three months of age. He cried often—screamed, really—had red patches on his cheeks and buttocks, was extremely irritable and difficult to handle, and had frequent diarrhea. She was angry that her pediatrician refused to do skin tests on the boy or give him what she called "nerve" pills, presumably to calm the baby.

By the time he was twelve months old, he had been on what Carol called a "milk-free" diet. One evening I ran into Carol and her baby in the local supermarket. He was having a tantrum and was squirming to get out of the grocery cart. His cheeks were bright red, with visible crusty areas. His eyelids were swollen and surrounded by heavy, dark circles. She said that he was miserable because he had a nasty diaper rash. Still, she was "very happy to run into me" so that she could ask me which ice cream I would recommend she serve at her baby's first birthday party. I asked her, "Why are you giving him ice cream?" To which she answered strongly, "I will not deny him ice cream and cake on his birthday!" At that point, when I saw how miserable this baby looked physically and how miserably he acted emotionally, I wondered how many other allergens his mother refused to deny him and how many other instructions from her baby's pediatrician she chose to ignore. Clearly, this mother needed to learn more about her baby's medical condition and the medical treatments that were appropriate for him. She also needed to learn more about her role as a nurturer and to respect the potential danger she was subjecting her baby to by not feeding him properly.

The point is, there are two health worlds in your dairy-sensitive child's life: the magical world of medicine and the real world of food, family, and nutrition. These work best in combination to promote healthy kids. Understanding both of these worlds will make you a better parent and your child a healthier and happier person. This chapter is devoted to the world of medicine, a world in which parents, even though they may not be trained doctors or pharmacists, need some sophistication in order to make over-the-counter medication purchases wisely and to assist their child's pediatrician and pharmacist in prescribing medications and treatments appropriately.

Prescription Drugs

In 1938, the U.S. Food, Drug, and Cosmetic Act required that all drugs introduced after that date must be safe for human use. In 1951, an amendment to the act mandated prescriptions for all drugs that could only be taken safely with medical supervision. Included in this classification were drugs that could be habit-forming, toxic, potentially harmful or were new and unproven. All the rest were sold over the counter. In 1962, additional amendments to the act required that all drug ingredients be proven effective for their intended uses. This requirement only pertained to prescription drugs and not to over-the-counter drugs at all. However, in 1972, the FDA instituted an extensive over-the-counter drug review program meant to ensure that all drugs contained in both prescription and over-the-counter remedies are both safe and effective for their intended purposes.

There has been some controversy surrounding these FDA panels. If parents are interested in learning more about drugs that are on the market, but contain ingredients that have been deemed ineffective, there are a number of sources to consult. The first place to start is the Public Citizen Health Research Group. Consult the appendix for more information.

Physicians are taught to dispense drugs under the rule of the "five Rs," meaning the right drug for the right patient in the right dose by the right route at the right time. Physicians prescribe drugs with the help of their patients. The patient offers a complete medical history; a detailed description of symptoms, which leads to the correct diagnosis; a history of allergic reactions to drugs taken in the past; and details of other chronic health problems, which may affect the choice of the prescription drug therapy. Parents must take responsibility for good communication with their child's physician regarding the details of their child's health history. Parents of dairy-sensitive children, therefore, must always remember to remind their child's physician of his or her milk-protein allergy or lactose intolerance. It could make a difference in a physician's choice of prescribed drugs.

All prescription drugs have instructions on the label for taking and storing the medicine. There may be other instructions included as well, such as the reason the medicine was prescribed (name of illness), how it works to help the illness, a few explanatory facts about the illness, and a list of potential side effects. These days, with the advent of widespread computer technology in the pharmacy, patients may be given a brochure to read that contains a wealth of helpful information.

While you do have to be a physician or pharmacist to dispense a prescription, you don't have to be a physician or pharmacist to read one. Most of the symbols and phrases doctors use to write prescriptions are abbreviated Latin or Greek words, holdovers from the days when doctors actually did write prescriptions in Latin. For example, the word "bid" is a shortened version of the Latin phrase, *bis in die,* meaning twice a day. Some other often-seen words and abbreviations on prescriptions are A2, meaning "both ears"; ac, meaning "before meals"; qd, meaning "once a day"; and Sig, which stands for "label as follows."

The number of pills or capsules prescribed is denoted by the symbol #. Table 8.1 lists many more prescription phrases that will help you interpret other directions to the pharmacist.

Even so, you will probably have some questions for the pharmacist. For example, the prescription might read, "two teaspoons every four hours." Does that mean you should wake your baby every four hours to give the medication? In some cases, the answer will be yes, in other cases, the answer will be no. The prescription may require that food or milk be taken. Does that mean to give the food or milk before or after giving your child the medicine? If your child cannot take any milk, will juice suffice? Within what time frame should your child be given the food? Are there foods your child should not be given while on this medication? Should your child continue to take the medication even after he or she feels better? Your pharmacist is an important source of information and may be consulted after you get home or at any time during the length of your child's illness.

It is imperative that you inform your pharmacist of your child's milk allergy or lactose intolerance. Many prescription drugs contain milk derivatives, especially lactose, and if the medication will make your child sicker, your physician might want to choose another medication. Later in this chapter, you will learn more about lactose in drugs and discover which ones to avoid, if possible.

Your pharmacist may also be able to help you give your child prescription drugs more effectively through a variety of measuring and dispensing aids. For example, if the prescription reads "two teaspoons," everyday silverware is not an appropriate dispenser. The teaspoon measurement must be exact and using any old small spoon in the drawer will not do. A standard measuring spoon may be used, or you may wish to use one of the combination measuring/dispensing utensils that make giving liquid medicine to children extremely easy. Your pharmacist can also help you explore ways to get the medicine down comfortably if your child balks. All parents have their favorite method: Some instruct their children to hold their nose to kill the flavor or offer rewards for speedy swallowing. Some medications can be mixed with fruit juice or other foods such as applesauce for easy dispensing. Children who can swallow pills might do best if they drink a few big gulps of lemonade or fruit punch to wash the pills down. In some cases, however, only water may be permitted. In this case, parents might want to reward their child with a frozen juice pop fifteen or twenty minutes later. Always check with your physician or pharmacist for the proper dispensing procedure.

Before giving your child medication, try to obtain the answers to all of the following questions:

1. What is the name of the drug?
2. What will this drug do to help my child?
3. How many days should the drug be given?
4. How should the drug be given—with water, juice, on an empty stomach, with food?
5. Should the drug be taken by mouth, rectally, or in the nose, eyes, or ears?
6. What foods or drinks should my child avoid while on the medication?
7. Should any of my child's activities be curtailed while taking the medication?
8. Are there other medications my child should avoid while taking this drug?
9. What side effects can we expect? Is there anything to do to help curtail the possibility of side effects?
10. Does the medication contain lactose?
11. Does the medication contain casein or another milk protein?
12. Should the drug be taken during the night?
13. How should the drug be stored?

Never give your child a drug prescribed for another child or for an adult. Only give prescriptions drugs to your child that have been specifically formulated for his or her weight, age, diagnosed illnesses, and medical appropriateness.

Table 8.1 Reading Your Child's Prescription:
Some Common Symbols and Their Meanings

ABBREVIATION	MEANING
A2	both ears
ac	before meals
AD	right ear
AL	left ear
AM	morning
AS	left ear
bid	twice a day
cap	capsule
disp	dispense
dtd#	give this number
ext	for external use
gtts	drops
HS	bedtime
mitt#	give this number
O2	both eyes
OD	right eye
OL	left eye
OU	each eye
pc	after meals
po	by mouth
prn	as needed
qd	once a day
qid	four times a day

ABBREVIATION	MEANING
qod	every other day
sl	under the tongue
tid	three times a day
top	apply topically
UT	under the tongue
ut dict	as directed
x	times

Filling Prescriptions

Your physician will prescribe the total amount of medication necessary for your child's treatment. However, that does not mean you are required to have the pharmacist fill the entire prescription at once. Drugs are not returnable. Therefore, especially if your child has had a bad reaction to a drug in the past, you may want to purchase only a couple of days' worth of the drug in order to make sure it is received well by your child. By doing this, if your child develops an allergic reaction or a stomach upset or some other side effect requiring the prescription to be changed, you haven't wasted the medication or the money you spent to purchase it. Always make sure first, however, that the remaining amount of medication will be available to your child when it is needed.

There may be other reasons you might want a partial prescription. For one, the drug could be very expensive, and, if your child will be taking it for an extended period of time, filling the prescription only partially would enable you to pay for it in increments. However, you should check this practice with your insurance company if you have one that helps with prescription drugs. Find out whether each incremental filling of the prescription requires a minimum payment; this might eventually add up to more than you thought.

If the drug is one your child will be taking over a long period of time, say over the course of several months, you might be able to purchase it in large quantities that will save you money. Always make sure you have enough of the medications your child needs for those times when you travel or during holiday periods when the pharmacy might be closed or for other special situations like summer camp, overnight stays with friends, and scout trips. In some situations, serious side effects could occur if children who need prescribed doses of medication have their treatment schedule interrupted.

Most importantly, keep a record. Each child (and each parent, for that matter) should have his or her own home medical record noting the date of the illness, the name of the illness, the medication prescribed, and the side effects, if any, that occur. This will be a valuable record of your child's health, especially if your family moves or switches medical caregivers, or changes health insurance companies.

Storing Medications

Some medications may lose their potency if they are not protected from heat or moisture. Usually prescription drugs may be stored safely at room temperature out of direct sunlight. Contrary to what most people think, prescription drugs generally should not be kept in warm, moist bathrooms. A medicine cabinet, safely out of reach of your child, could be in the den or the bedroom where there is no shower or bathtub. Keep all medications out of direct sunlight at all times, regardless of the packaging. It does not matter if the bottle or container is a dark color.

Some drugs require refrigeration, but this does not mean they may be frozen. A medication that requires a cold atmosphere must be kept in the refrigerator and protected from any extremely

---

Ideal Storage Temperatures for Medication

Cold—under 46° Fahrenheit

Refrigerator—between 36° and 46° Fahrenheit

Cool—between 46° and 59° Fahrenheit

Room Temperature—between 59° and 86° Fahrenheit

Excessive Heat—above 104° Fahrenheit

---

cold section where it might freeze accidentally. Some liquid medications, if frozen, separate into layers that cannot be remixed, or they might become so thick they will not pour out of the bottle. Some capsules or coated tablets might crack in the freezer.

Always remember to flush unwanted medications down the toilet or pour leftover liquids down the sink. Check your child's prescription for an expiration date. Regularly clean out the medicine cabinet and always keep it locked when you have small, curious children about.

Generic Drugs

Every new drug must undergo clinical investigation before it is released to the public, and during this time it is given a generic name by the United States Adopted Names Council, which is an organization sponsored by the American Medical Association. The generic name is usually a simplified version of the chemical formulation of the drug. When the drug has been deemed safe and effective by the FDA, it is ready for marketing. The pharmaceutical company producing the drug now gives it a brand name and registers that name as a trademark. The patent obtained by the pharmaceutical company for the drug gives the company exclusive rights to production and sales, usually for the next seventeen years. At that time, other manufacturers may begin producing the drug under its generic name. Until then, however, even if the physician prescribes the drug by its generic name, it may only be filled by the brand-name product.

Once the patent expires, and the drug can be manufactured by other companies, competition sets in and the price falls. In fact, brand-name drugs are usually five to ten times and sometimes up to thirty times more expensive than their generic counterparts. Some people assume that brand-name drugs are manufactured by the bigger, better companies, and generics are only manufactured by the smaller, inferior companies. This is simply not true. All prescription drugs marketed in the United States are monitored by the FDA, and there have been examples of both types of preparations, generic and brand-name, which have been cited for lack of efficacy or for other problems due to problems in the manufacturing process, regardless of whether the manufacturer was a large company or a small one. Basically, if the chemical formulation is the same, which it must be according to our present laws, all generic drugs are as safe and effective as the comparable brand-name drugs.

Often, the biggest difference between generic and brand-name drugs is in advertising and promotion. Remember that the pharmaceutical companies want doctors and pharmacists to recommend their product to patients and customers, and they spend enormous amounts of money to advertise those products in professional journals. The drug companies give out huge quantities of free samples for physicians to dispense to their patients. They sponsor conferences and educational trips for health-care professionals, and they even give cash awards to physicians and pharmacists for prescribing their drugs or selling their over-the-counter products. Naturally these practices translate into higher prices for consumers.

As managed care insurance programs come to dominate the health-care industry, parents will often be required to purchase a generic drug for their child. Managed care programs, including health maintenance organizations (HMOs), are based on the premise that the most expensive health-care practices do not necessarily yield the highest quality results. Higher costs may just mean waste or overinflated profits for pharmaceutical companies or other medical industry constituents. Even if your insurance company does not require that you purchase generic drugs, you still may want to check to see if a generic is available in order to save money on your own. You should let your child's pediatrician know that you want to have a generic drug prescribed whenever possible, and also inform your pharmacist that you prefer to have all prescriptions filled with generic drugs if available.

Over-the-Counter Drugs

Thousands of medicines are available without a prescription, although this in no way diminishes the caution parents should exercise when giving drugs to their children. Remember that even everyday drugs such as aspirin or acetaminophen can be toxic. Over-the-counter drugs have been determined to be safe, if taken as recommended, and have no restrictions on the amounts that may be purchased or on the identity of the buyer or the vendor. Over-the-counter drugs may be sold in supermarkets, candy stores, bus stations, or even summer camps.

Over-the-counter drugs may be highly effective for myriad illnesses and allergies. The experts in the field of over-the-counter drugs are generally pharmacists, who monitor the effect of such preparations among their customers. For example, if your physician has prescribed baby aspirin for your child, you would do well to check with your pharmacist about the various brands available. Ask if there has been feedback from other customers about these products. Some may report that one particular brand is more palatable than another. Sometimes it's a minor detail that could matter to you; you may be glad to learn that a particular brand of baby aspirin stains clothes if it is spit back up. Your pharmacist should be able to share some helpful information with you and help you make wise choices.

Your pharmacist should also keep a record of all the drugs your baby or child takes and should warn you of possible harmful interactions that could occur even among over-the-counter medications. Always remind your pharmacist of your child's dairy sensitivity and ask him or her to double check the ingredients in the medication you choose so that you can avoid dairy by-products if necessary.

Ask a lot of questions in the pharmacy. You need to know that if your child is being given the antibiotic tetracycline, for example, that it will negatively react with other iron-containing products, such as the over-the-counter vitamin and mineral supplement your child takes. But you might be able to avoid a problem if you separate the tetracycline and the iron preparation by at least two hours. It is the pharmacist's job to guide you and help you properly dispense medications to your child for the optimum benefit, so feel free to communicate with the pharmacist regularly.

Hidden Dangers in the Pharmacy for the Dairy-Sensitive Child

There are important differences in drugs that you should be aware of. These differences occur regardless of whether or not the drug is a brand name or a generic, a prescription drug or an over-the-counter preparation. There are a variety of hidden dangers for dairy-sensitive children, not the least of which are found in the inert ingredients used in the manufacture of drugs, and these will vary from company to company. Drugs contain inactive ingredients, defined as those which potentially have no physiological actions. They include stabilizers, colors, binders, sugars, and flavors. There may also be additional medically inactive ingredients such as caffeine included in the medicine you buy. But as you well know, many of these so-called inactive ingredients can cause potentially serious difficulties for sensitive children.

Parents of allergic children will have to be on the lookout for dangers to their children. These may include corn or soy or milk derivatives and may cause allergic reactions or diarrhea.

One pharmaceutical organization that may provide you with some help is the Professional Compounding Centers of America or PCCA. They can give you a list of pharmacies or specific pharmacists in your area able to formulate your allergic child's medications on a custom basis, thereby eliminating specific inactive ingredients that your child is allergic to, such as corn starch or red dyes. The phone number for the PCCA is 1-800-331-2498. There may also be pharmacies capable of formulating hypoallergenic drugs that can be shipped to you, in case you are not near any of the custom pharmacies. Obviously, this will be difficult for prescriptions needed immediately.

Parents of lactose-intolerant children have an even greater challenge in the pharmacy. That's because lactose is used as a binder in literally thousands of prescription drugs and over-the-counter preparations. It is also used in liquid medications to add some sweetness without adding sucrose. You may even find lactose in drugs prescribed for your child's diarrhea, even though taking the medication with lactose could cause more diarrhea.

Basically, there are two ways of dealing with lactose in medications. One is to ask for a replacement drug that is manufactured without lactose. Your pharmacist will probably work together with your child's pediatrician to make another selection. Or, you may have to do the research yourself. A variety of resources are available to you in the library such as the *Physician's Desk Reference,* or drug information books published by the American Family Health Institute or the editors of *Consumer Guide* or the Public Citizen Health Research Group. You may have to go to the library and obtain phone numbers of various pharmaceutical manufacturers and make some calls yourself to see if lactose or other offensive ingredients are in the medications prescribed for your child.

You cannot always rely on the label for complete information either. A complete list of ingredients is not required by law on pharmaceutical preparations. It is also true that there may not be complete disclosure in sourcebooks that list medications, their purposes, active and inactive ingredients, and contraindications. This includes the *Physician's Desk Reference* books. Complete ingredient disclosure is provided by the drug companies on a voluntary basis. However, the Pharmaceutical Manufacturers Association, the Generic Pharmaceutical Industry Association, and the Propriety Association—all groups that include the majority of drug suppliers in this country—have made a commitment to complete ingredient disclosure. Therefore, especially in the last five years, we have seen more ingredient information on drug labels than ever before.

I hope that the trend will continue. Years ago, many drug companies would not even answer specific inquiries about ingredients from the general public. In 1980, when I was doing research for my first book, I could only get complete ingredient information from some pharmaceutical companies through one of my friends, who was a physician. That, too, is changing. While you may bump up against a few roadblocks in this area, generally you will be able to determine whether there are any ingredients in your child's medication that will prompt an allergic reaction or a bout of digestive distress.

The second way to handle lactose in medications is to give your lactose-intolerant child lactase enzyme supplements just before taking the medication. The enzymes may be very helpful, because the amount of lactose present in medicine is usually small, compared to say, a half a glass of milk. Using enzyme supplements could be quite important for your child, especially if no lactose-free drug preparation is available. I would recommend calling the enzyme supplement company to obtain information about the best way to use supplements along with medications. And don't settle for speaking to a person who cannot answer your question. If the person who answers the phone does not know the answer, ask to speak with someone else. If the enzyme supplement company cannot give you adequate information about its product, choose another supplement from a company that conducts its own research.

Table 8.2 lists a number of drugs that contain lactose. As with all lists of this kind, it may not be completely up to date, as manufactured drug preparations change quickly. Always double check for lactose with the physician, pharmacist, or drug manufacturer. Remember that thousands of drugs are manufactured in this country and this list only represents a handful of them.

Selecting a Lactase Enzyme Supplement

Several companies, large and small, have been in the business of producing lactase enzyme supplements for many, many years. Over the past five years, however, the industry has grown enormously due to an increase in the number of Americans diagnosed with lactose intolerance and the desire of pharmaceutical companies to capture this market. Pharmaceutical companies like McNeil Consumer Products Co., a division of Johnson and Johnson, manufactures Lactaid products. Its nearest competitor, Dairy Ease, is made by Miles Inc. Kremers-Urban pharmaceutical company is another well-known lactase enzyme product manufacturer, having produced Lactrase tablets and capsules for years. According to the *Wall Street Journal,* sales of lactase enzyme products soar above the $100 million mark yearly. This growing market has spawned the production and distribution of lactase enzyme supplements by several small, even very tiny, companies hoping to cash in on what they perceive to be a hot commodity.

What this means for the consumer, then, is that there are lots of choices in the marketplace for lactase enzyme supplements. Understand that the enzyme is usually derived from yeast or fungal sources and may be sold as chewable tablets, liquid, or in capsule form. In my research, I have come across a variety of scientific studies that have confirmed the relative effectiveness of lactase enzyme therapy using several products currently in the marketplace such as Lactaid and Lactrase. These are studies comparing these products, favoring one over another. But I have also read reports of various recalls of one batch of enzyme supplement or another; this is not terribly unusual because the efficacy of the supplements may be affected by a variety of factors, including heat and moisture. Therefore, it is certainly possible that even the best product does not perform at its peak all the time. Also note that conditions in the body—highly changeable and subjective—can affect the efficacy of the enzyme.

A study published in the journal *Digestive Diseases and Sciences,* November 1993, compared the effects of three popular lactase preparations, Lactaid caplet, Dairy Ease chewable tablet, and Lactogest soft gel capsule. The study found that all three enzyme preparations dramatically reduced both the peak and total breath hydrogen production when the subjects were fed a portion of milk containing 20 g of lactose. Four capsules of Lactogest, two caplets of Lactaid, or two tablets of Dairy Ease were used to achieve these results. However, when 50 g of lactose was ingested, the peak and total hydrogen production was only modestly, not significantly, reduced by the enzyme treatment. Furthermore, symptom scores for bloating, cramping, nausea, pain, diarrhea, and flatus were not different between treatments. The unusually large dose of lactose (equivalent to about three to four cups of milk) appeared to overwhelm the ability of any of these products to comfortably reduce the symptoms of lactose intolerance. They all performed about the same.

Be aware that good products may be produced in bad batches occasionally. *Food Chemical News* of April 20, 1992, reported the recall of a batch of Dairy Ease liquid in 7 ml bottles because of the "subpotency" of the product's lactase enzyme. The nationwide recall was initiated in February 1992 by Sterling Drug Company. The manufacturer was Goto Shusei Ltd. of Tokyo, Japan. These things happen, so parents need to be on the lookout for the enzyme products in the quantities that seem to work best for their own children. But don't place unwavering faith in them.

I have been told by experts in the field, that enzymes which have been measured in Food Chemicals Codex Lactase Units (FCCLU) may be more reliable than those measured in simple milligrams. The FCCLU designation is assigned to an enzyme that has undergone testing for efficacy. In other words, the FCCLU designation measures the activity of the enzyme as opposed to a milligram (mg) designation, which only stands for quantity of the enzyme. For a list of some companies that produce enzyme supplements, please check the appendix.

Table 8.2 Some Medications That Contain Lactose

OVER-THE-COUNTER DRUGS	MANUFACTURER
Actifed Tablets	Warner Wellcome
Afrin Tablets	Schering-Plough
Allbee with C Caplets	A. H. Robins Company
Allbee C-800 Tablets	A. H. Robins Company
Allbee C-800 plus Iron Tablets	A. H. Robins Company
Allerest 12 Hour Caplets	Fisons Consumer Health
Bayer Enteric Aspirin	Sterling Winthrop
Bayer Delayed Release Enteric Aspirin	Sterling Winthrop
Benadryl 25 Tablets	Parke-Davis
Centrum High Potency Multivitamin	Lederle
Centrum Advanced from A-Zinc	Lederle
Centrum, Jr. (Children's Chewable)	Lederle
Chlor-Trimeton Allergy Tablets	Schering-Plough
Chlor-Trimeton 12 Hour Repetabs	Schering-Plough
Chlor-Trimeton Antihistamine and Decongestant Tablets	Schering-Plough
Chlor-Trimeton Non-Drowsy Decongestant Tablets	Schering-Plough
Contac Maximum Strength Continuous Action Nasal Decongestant Antihistamine Caplets	SmithKline Beecham

continues

OVER-THE-COUNTER DRUGS	MANUFACTURER
Drixoral Cold and Allergy Sustained-Action Tablets	Schering-Plough
Ex-Lax Chocolated Laxative Tablets	Sandoz
Guaitab Tablets	Muro
Hyland's Calms Forté Tablets	Standard Homeopathic
Hyland's Arnicaid Tablets	Standard Homeopathic
Hyland's C-Plus Cold Tablets	Standard Homeopathic
Hyland's EnurAid Tablets	Standard Homeopathic
Hyland's Teething Tablets	Standard Homeopathic
Hyland's Vitamin C for Children	Standard Homeopathic
Imodium A-D Caplets	McNeil
Nature's Remedy Natural Vegetable Laxative	SmithKline Beecham
Sleepinal Medicated Night Tea Packets	Thompson
Slow FE Tablets	Ciba
Sudafed Plus Tablets	Warner Wellcome
Tavist-D	Sandoz
Theragran Multivitamin Tablets	Bristol-Myers
Triaminic Cold Tablets	Sandoz
Triaminic-12 Tablets	Sandoz
Triaminicin Tablets	Sandoz
Triaminicol Multi-Symptom Cold Tablets	Sandoz
Unicap, Jr. Chewable Tablets	Upjohn

PRESCRIPTION DRUGS	MANUFACTURER
Ativan	Wyeth-Ayerst
Bumex	Roche
Capoten	Bristol-Myers Squibb
Catapres Tablets	Boehringer Ingelheim
Coumadin Tablets	Du Pont
Deltasone Tablets	Upjohn

PRESCRIPTION DRUGS	MANUFACTURER
Donnatal	A. H. Robins Company
Dyazide Capsules	SmithKline Beecham
E-Mycin Tablets	Boots
Eryc	Parke-Davis
Fiorinal	Sandoz
Flexeril Tablets	Merck
Glucotrol Tablets	Pratt
Hismanal Tablets	Janssen
IBU 800 Tablets	Boots
Inderal	Wyeth-Ayerst
Intal	Fisons
Macrodantin Capsules	Proctor & Gamble
Pen-Vee K Tablets	Wyeth-Ayerst
Phenergan	Wyeth-Ayerst
Restoril	Sandoz
Ritalin HCI	Ciba-Geigy
Seldane	Marion Merrell Dow
Seldane-D	Marion Merrell Dow
Sumycin	Apothecon
Synthroid	Boots
Theo-Dur	Key
Veetids	Apothecon
Xanax	Upjohn

Source: *American Druggist*, September 1993

Calcium-Robbing Drugs

One of the unfortunate side effects of some medications is the depletion of calcium stores in the body. This depletion occurs when medications interfere with calcium absorption or cause calcium to be released into the bloodstream, sweat, or urine. Parents need to be made aware of the possibility that their children's medication could be robbing their bodies of calcium. If this is the case, children might require calcium supplementation or perhaps a change to another medication. While calcium depletion may not be a problem if medicines are only taken occasionally, obviously this issue will be of greater concern for those children who take medications regularly, prophylactically, or over a long period of time. If your child is medicated regularly, you will want to discuss this issue with your child's pediatrician.

Calcium is closely regulated in the blood on a continuous basis so that the body has enough of the mineral to do whatever task is required. Only about 1 percent of the calcium in the body is circulated in the bloodstream, and this quantity is evenly maintained by hormones. The bloodstream will take calcium from minerals that are ingested or from the mineral stored in the bones. As you can imagine, your child must be taking in large amounts of calcium in order to do all the work required of his or her growing body, including storing calcium for use later in life. Recently, studies were done on two groups of children: One group took calcium supplements, and the other group was not supplemented. The results clearly indicated that those children who were supplemented had substantially greater bone density than the others. Greater bone density provides clear protection against devastating bone loss later in life.

Because dairy-sensitive children are already limited in their ability to ingest high calcium dairy foods, the last thing parents want to do is to sabotage their good efforts to provide adequate calcium intake for their children by giving them medicines that deplete their children's calcium stores. But sometimes it cannot be helped. In that case, parents need to be aware of the situation and supplement their child's diet with calcium accordingly. Also, please do not let yourself be put off by a physician or nurse who might insist that your child is perfectly fine because his blood levels of calcium are okay. Calcium levels in the blood do not reflect calcium stores in the bones. If your child is taking one or more of the calcium-robbing drugs on a regular basis, you are going to need better counseling than that.

It is important that you provide an atmosphere at home that is conducive to your child absorbing the calcium he or she does ingest. Limit caffeine and soda pop. Both of these interfere with calcium absorption. Parents hope their children will not smoke, but do be aware that smoking also interferes with calcium absorption. This includes secondhand smoke. Weight-bearing exercise enhances bone density, so encourage your child to run and jump and dance and climb.

Recently, the National Osteoporosis Foundation launched a campaign to raise awareness of the role prescription drugs play in interfering with calcium absorption. The drugs in question include glucocorticoids, such as cortisone, hydrocortisone, prednisone, prednisolone, dexamethasone, betamethasone,

---

Brand Names of Drugs That May Interfere with Calcium Absorption

Ak-Cide	Inflamase
Ak-Dex	Inflamase Forte
Ak-Tate	Maxidrex
Beclovent	Nova-Pred
Decaderm	Novoprednisolone
Decadron	Pred Forte
Decadron LA	Pred-G
Delta-Cortef	Pred Mile
Deronil	Prelone
Dexasone	Propaderm
Dexone	Vanceril
Hexadrol	

flunisolide, and beclomethasone dipropionate. These drugs are prescribed for the treatment of arthritis, asthma, allergies, ulcerative colitis, liver disease, lupus, cancer, and organ transplants.

Anticonvulsants such as phenytoin and barbiturates used to control epileptic seizures and heart problems have also been shown to cause bone wasting. Likewise, children who are given large amounts of aluminum-based antacids (like Maalox, Rolaids, Gelusil, Gaviscon, and others) are at increased risk for bone loss. Other drugs that have the same negative effect include methotrexate, used to fight cancer and other immune disorders including arthritis, and cyclosporin A, used to protect organ transplants and also used in some cases of Crohn's disease and insulin-dependent diabetes. Some of the brand names in these categories are listed below.

Brand Names of Drugs That May Cause Bone Wasting

Barbidonna	Luminal
Barbidonna Elixir	Mebroin
Barbita	Mexate
Belladenal	Mundrane GG Elixir and Tablets
Bellergal	
Bronchotabs	Neuro-Spasex
Chardonna	Neuro-Transentin
Diclophen	Neuro-Transentin Forte
Dilantin	Phenaphen
Dilantin with Phenobarbitol	Phenergan VC with Codeine
Diphenylan	Quadrinal
Folex	Sandimunne
Gardenal	Solfoton
Kinesed	Tedral

Naturally, if your child is taking any one of these medications, it is because he or she is dealing with health problems quite out of the ordinary. He or she is surely being monitored closely by a physician. Please speak to your physician about this information and continue to do your very best to ensure that your growing child or teenager is adequately supplied with the calcium needed for lifelong good health.

Common Types of Medication Given to Children—A Glossary of Terms

Analgesics Drugs used to relieve pain. Some are narcotic, derived from the opium poppy and act on the brain to cause deep analgesia and often drowsiness. Narcotics give the patient a feeling of well-being and are addictive. Nonnarcotic analgesics are most commonly derived from salicylates such as aspirin. Acetaminophen is another example of a nonnarcotic pain reliever, although it does not act on inflammation like aspirin. Both aspirin and acetaminophen are effective in reducing a child's temperature from a fever, but certain childhood illnesses require the use of one or the other. They are not always interchangeable.

Anthelmintics Drugs used to treat worm infestations.

Antibacterials Drugs used to treat many bacterial infections.

Antibiotics Special kinds of antibacterials derived from molds or produced synthetically. Antibiotics destroy or inhibit the growth of bacteria and fungi, but do not counteract viruses. Must be taken for a specified period of time, even after the child seems to feel better, in order to ensure that the infection is completely resolved. Otherwise, the bacterial infection could reappear or resistant bacteria could emerge.

Anticholinergics Used to slow the action of the bowel and reduce the amount of stomach acid. Sometimes referred to as antispasmodics.

Anticonvulsants These drugs are used to control most symptoms of epilepsy by selectively reducing excessive stimulation in the brain.

Antidiarrheals These may be narcotic or nonnarcotic medications used to slow the action of the bowel to check diarrhea. Some antidiarrheals are available over the counter and others are only available by prescription.

Antifungals Drugs used to treat infections caused by fungi.

Antihistamines Drugs used to block the effects of histamine, a chemical released in the body after an allergic reaction. This usually causes swelling and itching. Some antihistamines cause drowsiness, others do not. Severe histamine reactions may require the use of an injectable epinephrine, administered either on-site, in case of an emergency, or at the physician's office or hospital.

Anti-inflammatories Medications used to reduce inflammation or swelling and the symptoms of inflammation such as pain, fever, redness, and itching. Aspirin is an anti-inflammatory drug. So are ibuprofen and naproxyn. Steroids are also used to treat such inflammatory diseases as Crohn's, arthritis, or asthma.

Antinauseants Drugs used to reduce the urge to vomit. They may be administered orally, rectally, or intravenously.

Antitussives These drugs control coughs and may be either narcotic or nonnarcotic. They must circulate through the brain before they act on a cough and therefore must be taken with water.

Antivirals Drugs used to combat viral infections.

Bronchodilators   Agents that relax airways in the lungs or relax smooth muscle tissue such as that found in the lungs. Used in the treatment of asthma or emphysema.

Chemotherapeutics   Synthetically produced drugs used to treat various types of infections or cancer.

Decongestants   Drugs that constrict the blood vessels in the nose and sinuses to open up air passages. May be taken orally or through nose drops or sprays. Oral decongestants are slow-acting and do not interfere with the production of mucus. They do increase blood pressure. Nose drops or sprays provide almost immediate relief and do not increase blood pressure as much as the others. These products may become ineffective after time.

Expectorants   Medications that are supposed to bring up phlegm through coughing, although their effectiveness is controversial. Often drinking water or using a vaporizer or humidifier may be equally effective or more effective in expectorating mucus through coughing.

Insulin   A hormone secreted by the pancreas that regulates the level of sugar in the blood and the metabolism of carbohydrates and fats.

Local anesthetics   Anesthetics applied directly to a painful area for such problems as toothaches or earaches.

Pediculicides   Drugs used to treat lice.

Scabicides   Drug used to treat scabies.

Sedatives   Drugs that have a calming effect, used to treat anxiety or insomnia.

Steroids   Steroids are found naturally in the body, as a result of the pituitary gland hormone ACTH, or may be produced synthetically. The function of steroids is anti-inflammatory. They may be administered orally for diseases of the immune system or administered topically for the treatment of hives, insect bites, or poison ivy.

Topical dermatologics   Drugs used to treat a variety of skin disorders ranging from dry skin to acne. Skin disorders are usually treated most effectively with prescription drugs.

Tranquilizers   These drugs calm certain areas of the brain but permit the rest of the brain to function normally. They act as a screen that allows transmission of some nerve impulses while restricting others.

Vaccines   These are serums containing weakened or dead disease-causing microorganisms, which activate the body to develop a natural immunity against a particular disease such as polio or measles.

9

Ouch!
My Tummy Hurts!

Homespun remedies to cure diarrhea have been passed on from generation to generation the world over. No doubt, your family has its favorite method of treating this painful and distressing condition. And as surely as folk remedies have been treasured throughout the centuries, if you are the parents of a dairy-sensitive child who gets diarrhea, you will be given more than your fair share of advice in this area.

Trust me. Everyone has an antidiarrhea remedy—your mother, your best friend, your child's nursery school teacher. In a book called *Chicken Soup & Other Folk Remedies,* Joan and Lydia Wilen report that the favorite cure for diarrhea since biblical times has been the common blackberry. Apparently, people have believed that blackberry juice or blackberry brandy given every four hours will do the trick. Other favorite folk remedies include feeding scraped apple, and nothing but scraped apple, until the condition subsides; drinking water every other hour in which rice has been boiled (preferably brown rice); eating cooked rice with a dash of cinnamon; eating bananas to "promote the growth of beneficial bacteria in the intestine"; or adding one teaspoonful of finely chopped garlic to one teaspoonful of honey taken three times a day, two hours after each meal. Trust me again, none of these remedies are appropriate for your infant, toddler, child, or teenager. Do not give garlic and honey, sauerkraut juice, pickled beets, pickled cucumbers, raw sauerkraut, kefir, or buttermilk to your child thinking that any of these will cure his or her diarrhea.

Diarrhea has been studied by scientists very carefully because diarrhea is not a folksy condition calling for a folksy cure. Diarrhea kills children all over the world—yes, even in America—and must be handled carefully and properly by parents whose children suffer with it. While it may not be a proper topic for dinner-table conversation, the subject of diarrhea must be addressed because sooner or later your child will have it.

The best place I can think of to discuss diarrhea is right here, in a book devoted to answering your questions about raising children without milk. No matter what the cause, milk is the last thing you want to ever give a child suffering with a bout of diarrhea. For proven remedies, we will consult the experts, pediatricians and other scientists who have studied diarrhea and have developed solutions to the health problems that accompany this potentially serious and possibly life-threatening medical condition.

According to the *Tufts University Diet & Nutrition Letter,* at least one child per day is killed in the United States by diarrhea. Usually it is a baby under twelve months old. More than five hundred children per day are hospitalized for diarrhea, amounting to more than 200,000 hospital admissions every year and costing the nation's health-care system more than $500 million annually. The Centers for Disease Control has reportedly expressed concern about these statistics, because, in its view, many of these hospitalizations have been deemed "preventable."

In response, several national health organizations have worked together to launch what is known as the National Oral Rehydration Project. Through this project, parents and health-care professionals are offered educational materials, seminars, and workshops that explain easy and inexpensive methods of preventing a case of diarrhea from developing into a life-threatening situation. The goal of the program is to encourage parents especially to always keep a supply of an oral rehydration solution in the home to be given to a child during a bout of serious diarrhea. The rehydration formula may taste like fruit juice, but it is a substantially different beverage and should be respected just as a parent would respect a poison antidote like syrup of ipecac, for example.

To understand the importance of keeping this specially formulated rehydration solution in the home at all times, first you must understand a bit about diarrhea itself. When the body is functioning properly, there is a normal balance of water in the stool. When diarrhea strikes, extra water stores are called to the bowel from other areas of the body and the stool becomes loose—full of extra water. As the diarrhea moves very quickly through the colon, all of the water, including the excess, is excreted. When the body loses too much water, it becomes dehydrated, a condition that is especially dangerous for babies and, incidentally, older people as well. And water isn't the only thing that diarrhea takes with it. It takes minerals such as potassium and sodium. These minerals in proper balance are essential to life itself, and herein lies the problem.

Ordinary, self-limiting diarrhea is one thing. But severe or prolonged diarrhea will threaten life by dehydrating the body and upsetting the balance of the life-giving minerals called electrolytes. Electrolytes in the body are ionized salts, including sodium, potassium, and chlorine, that act as conductors of electric impulses in the blood, tissue fluids, and cells. The proper balance of these components is essential to the functioning of blood, tissue fluids, and cells—in other words, essential to life itself.

To avoid the loss of electrolytes, it is imperative that rehydration (putting liquids back into the body) takes place during a bout of diarrhea. Sometimes if the diarrhea is mild, giving children much more water than usual is enough. But occasionally, if the diarrhea is severe, your pediatrician will recommend giving the child an oral rehydration solution that has been specially formulated to replace vital minerals and other nutrients (electrolytes) that have been lost. You can see, then, why, in some cases, juice or rice water is simply inadequate. You can also see why, if your child is an infant and is suffering severely, having the rehydration formula on hand will be extremely helpful in case it is required during the middle of the night or after store hours.

Oral rehydration solutions are available in supermarkets, pharmacies, and discount stores, really anywhere that infant formula is found. They may be available in a powder form, to which water must be added, or already mixed in bottles. Trade names include Lytren, Resol, Pedialyte, and Infalyte. They are available in a variety of flavors including fruit and bubble gum.

Your child's pediatrician will instruct you in the proper method of administering an oral rehydration solution, based on your child's age, weight, and the nature of the diarrhea. Usually, infants or other very young children will be given small amounts frequently, such as two teaspoons every two to three minutes, or about one cup altogether in between episodes of diarrhea. Naturally, this involves plenty of patience on your part, but is worth it if hospitalization can be avoided. If your child is under two years old, your pediatrician will want to be called frequently and kept apprised of the situation. It is recommended that if the diarrhea gets worse or continues for longer than twenty-four hours, the physician should be called, no matter how old the child is. These rehydration solutions are all free of lactose and milk proteins and may therefore be administered to all children, regardless of their dairy sensitivity.

During a bout of diarrhea, it is important to note the frequency of your child's urination and the color of the urine as well. If the urine is unusually dark, this must be reported to the physician since it probably means that too much water is passing through the bowel and not enough is reaching the kidneys to form urine that will properly dilute the waste it carries away. All liquids, whether water, juice, or rehydration solution, may be given again after the child spits up or vomits. In fact, dehydration can actually cause vomiting, so giving more and more fluids may help the vomiting resolve as well. Don't worry about giving your child too much liquid. He needs more than usual now.

There is some controversy over feeding regular foods during a bout of diarrhea. Some parents are advised to take their children off solid foods for at least twenty-four hours in order to give the bowel a chance "to rest." This regimen is recommended by T. Berry Brazelton, M.D., noted pediatrician practicing at Children's Hospital in Boston and professor of pediatrics at Harvard Medical School. According to Brazelton in his book *Touchpoints,* the child's "digestive system needs to rest, so give her only foods that can be absorbed easily. Clear liquids—broth, sweet tea, flat ginger ale, or diluted clear juices like apple juice— are best." He also instructs parents to ignore the problem of a re- cently toilet-trained child needing diapers again. His advice about diapers is "Just offer them; don't make a fuss."

However, some studies have suggested that withholding food may not be helpful in the treatment of diarrhea. In fact, these studies have shown that the sooner the child is fed, the less severe the diarrhea will be and the sooner it will end. This regi- men is the one preferred by Dr. Benjamin Spock in his recently updated book *Dr. Spock's Baby and Child Care.* He explains, "It used to be that a baby with mild diarrhea would be taken off his solids and formula and instead given a lot of liquids that are high in sugar (such as gelatin water, soda, or apple juice). But now re- search has shown that this traditional 'diarrhea diet' actually in- creases and prolongs diarrhea. So for mild, brief infant diarrhea, offer breast milk or formula and the baby's regular diet, and let him eat as much as he seems hungry for. This is what works best." Obviously, you will have to consult your child's pediatrician for advice on this issue and determine for yourself what works best for your child.

What the preeminent pediatricians do agree on, however, is the treatment of severe diarrhea. But how do you know if your child's diarrhea is severe? According to Dr. Spock, severe diar- rhea is diarrhea that hasn't resolved in a couple of days, occurs markedly more often than the regular number of stools per day, or has pus or blood in it. He instructs parents, "If [your child] is vomiting, has fever, or seems generally ill, then you must contact your doctor or a hospital emergency room promptly." According to Dr. Brazelton, "Blood and mucus in the stool are danger signs. If you spot any or if severe diarrhea persists for more than twenty- four hours, call your doctor."

One common adult remedy, which is often recommended for the treatment of diarrhea, is rice water with honey. According to Dr. James E. Strain, clinical professor of pediatrics at the University of Colorado, this remedy may be fine for treating older children with mild diarrhea, but is not appropriate for severe diarrhea or for young babies who should never be given honey. Honey has been linked to cases of infant botulism. The best advice, then, is to avoid home remedies and instead stick to sensible feeding and whatever regimen is recommended by your child's pediatrician.

Please be aware that many over-the-counter medicines for the treatment of diarrhea should not be used on children. The World Health Organization (WHO) has recently published a report entitled "The Rational Use of Drugs in the Management of Acute Diarrhea in Children." After reviewing the efficacy and safety of the most often used antidiarrheal medications on the market, the authors of the report concluded, "Antidiarrheal drugs should never be used. None has any proven value and some are dangerous." The United States Centers for Disease Control and Prevention concurs with the recommendation of the WHO report.

Some consumer health groups are calling for a ban of these products in both prescription and over-the-counter forms, citing their potential dangerous side effects in children, including drowsiness and nausea and cessation of the function of the intestines. The pediatric prescription dosage forms of Lomotil, Imodium, Imodium A-D Liquid, and Pepto Diarrhea Control were singled out for unfavorable notice. The consumer groups have called for inclusion of a child's warning statement on the adult formulations of these drugs. Other drugs that were cited include Donnagel PG and other kaolin or pectin preparations. The report goes on to state that activated charcoal (Charcoal Plus, Charcocaps, and others) should not be used in the treatment of acute diarrhea in children either. However, its role in the treatment of poison ingestion is well documented; therefore, activated charcoal is not on the ban list.

Whether or not to give your child medication for his or her diarrhea is a subject you should discuss with your child's healthcare provider. But remember, most diarrhea is not severe and is therefore self-limiting. In other words, it will probably go away soon on its own.

Oral rehydration solutions are unanimously recommended for the treatment of acute diarrhea in children. According to the *Public Citizen Health Research Group Health Letter,* February 1993, "Management of diarrhea with ORS is considered one of the most important medical advances of this century. ORS is a simple, low-cost and easily obtainable method to prevent or correct the dehydration (the loss of body fluids and salts) that often accompanies diarrhea."

As you know, diarrhea will cause a secondary lactose intolerance, even in children who are not normally lactose intolerant. Therefore, milk or other dairy foods are always withheld during periods of diarrhea and recovery. This nondairy prescription is advisable for both children and adults.

Day-Care Diarrhea

Studies have shown that outbreaks of diarrhea in day-care centers are usually caused by a bacteria called *Shigella.* These bacteria are easily transmitted through contamination of diaper-changing areas. Children with this type of diarrhea need to be treated with antibiotics and usually do not return to day-care until stool cultures show that the infection is gone, which can take about one week. If your child is in a day-care center, you should check to make sure that proper hygiene is always practiced: This includes ensuring that caregivers wash their hands with soap and water after each stool diaper change. If your child goes to a day-care center and comes down with diarrhea, your child's pediatrician will probably want to run a stool culture to be certain of the cause. If an offending bacteria is found, antibiotics will need to be prescribed.

Toddler's Diarrhea— Apple Juice Diarrhea

Some children experience a type of chronic diarrhea although they are obviously thriving and seem to have no illness whatsoever. It may be referred to as "toddler's diarrhea" or "apple juice diarrhea." While their bowel movements may be normal at the beginning of the day, by the end of the day these children have loose or runny bowel movements. After being checked by the pediatrician, it may be determined that the child has a condition caused by too much sugar in the diet, particularly from drinking too much apple juice. In this situation, the child has ingested more carbohydrates than the enzymes necessary for digesting carbohydrates in the gut can handle. The solution is to cut back on the juice and sweets and see if the condition resolves itself.

Drugs That Exacerbate Diarrhea

The National Digestive Disease Information Clearinghouse has developed a number of fact sheets for the public giving information about various diseases or conditions that affect gastrointestinal health. One of the fact sheets is devoted to a discussion of medications that work against the gut. It is noted that diarrhea is often caused by antibiotics, which upset the natural intestinal balance of bacteria. Magnesium-based antacids may also cause diarrhea because they have a laxative effect. Laxatives need to be carefully administered so as not to produce diarrhea. For the child with lactose intolerance, or frequent diarrhea due to milk-protein allergy, any medication that exacerbates the occurrence of diarrhea will be a problem as will any medication manufactured with lactose as an inactive ingredient.

Comforting the Child with Diarrhea

Children with diarrhea will probably have some cramping and possibly some inflammation in the stomach or intestine. They will need to rest and might nap or sleep through the night longer than usual. They can be comforted with hugs, a warm hot-water bottle, a soothing drink, soft music, a favorite story, their blanket in the family room. They will need to be careful about bathroom hygiene and will probably require a little extra help cleaning themselves after evacuating. A warm shower or bath might also make the child feel better, in addition to cleaning her bottom. The child with diarrhea should wash his or her hands frequently to avoid spreading germs and so should the parent or baby-sitter caring for the child.

Infants may need extra periods of closeness including holding and rocking. The warmth of your body against the baby's body may act like a heating pad, soothing the tummy muscles. Don't worry about "spoiling" your child. (I *really* hate that word!) Your child is ill and needs more love and physical comforting to feel secure and help relieve the anxiety that accompanies her illness.

Simple Rules to Follow

If you are looking for a specific course of action to take when caring for your child with diarrhea, then let's take the best advice from the experts and follow this simple list of rules. These apply to the treatment of your baby or older child with diarrhea:

1. Contact the pediatrician for a proper diagnosis.
2. Begin ORS, oral rehydration solution, if advised to do so.
3. Eliminate all dairy foods for the duration of the condition.
4. Avoid caffeine (cola drinks, chocolate), which may stimulate the gut unnecessarily.

5. Offer your child plenty of water, juice, broth, and other clear liquids.

6. Be extra cautious about bathroom or diapering hygiene in order to avoid spreading germs.

7. Offer a light meal. Don't be afraid to feed your child if he or she is hungry.

8. Stay in contact with the pediatrician if the diarrhea gets worse or does not resolve quickly.

10   Sharing Your Thoughts with Other Parents

Raising children with allergies and food sensitivities can sometimes be an overwhelming task, but you will eventually, after many trials and many errors, come to rest upon an appropriate diet and lifestyle strategy for your child. I hope you will do so with the support and advice of excellent pediatricians, pediatric allergists, or pediatric gastroenterologists. In her book *Is This Your Child?*, Dr. Doris Rapp describes the feeling many parents get after learning about their children's food sensitivities and the sense of relief they often experience when their children are finally properly diagnosed and treated. Dr. Rapp writes, "Finding a major food that is causing your child to feel unwell or one that is contributing to your child's behavior or activity problems can be a tremendous relief. For the first time you realize that you are not a bad parent. Equally important, both you and your child will realize for the first time that your child is neither bad nor slow."

Dr. Penelope Leach, a psychologist and an expert in child development, in her book *Your Baby and Child from Birth to Age Five* discusses the importance of parents maintaining a good relationship with their children's health-care givers, while at the same time feeling confident enough to place equally great importance on their own understanding of their children. She maintains that parents, especially parents of allergic or food-intolerant children, must trust their child's pediatrician *and* themselves. She writes, "Rearing a child 'by the book'—by any set of rules or predetermined ideas—can work well if the rules you choose to follow fit the baby you happen to have." Leach suggests that parents should not necessarily do things "by the book," but rather "that you do them, always, 'by the baby.'" She goes on to say, "Bringing up a child in this flexible, thoughtful way takes time and effort. It involves extremely hard work as well as great rewards. But what worthwhile and creative job does not? Bringing up a child is one of the most creative, most worthwhile, and most undervalued of all jobs."

Dr. Leach also cautions parents of allergic and food-intolerant children not to be too hard on medical science. Over-vigilance in trying to hunt down allergens may not be in the best interest of the baby or child because science is limited in its ability to always identify allergens or substances causing intolerances. Besides, the process can often make a child and her family anxious, stressed, and overloaded by unanswerable questions. "Food allergies and intolerances are complex and often interrelated," writes Dr. Leach. "It is important not to leap to conclusions but to seek medical advice with an open mind, prepared to accept that there may not always be a simple solution to a problem and that it may take a long time to solve."

One of the most important lessons I learned as a parent of dairy-sensitive children was that sharing ideas and questions with other parents in the same situation is extremely helpful and emotionally rewarding. Who better to understand the nuances of precisely what you and your child may be going through than another parent experiencing a similar situation? Not that the other parent always has a correct answer to your question, but even so, together you can work to find the answer or compare notes on issues. It's like doing homework in a study group where three or four heads are definitely better than one. Someone may remember something you forgot or has tried a management solution that you might never have thought of but that could work well in your family.

In 1982, my first book about lactose intolerance and milk allergy was published (*Milk-Free Cookbook*). It was the culmination of all the research I had done at that time and all the effort I had made in the kitchen raising three dairy-sensitive children since the first was born in 1971. The response from others coping with dairy sensitivity was extremely welcome, and without exception, everyone who wrote me letters expressed great relief at finally having someone to talk to about dairy sensitivity who did not think they were crazy or suffering from hypochondriasis.

People feel great comfort when they realize they are not alone. I understand how they feel because I, too, am severely lactose intolerant, but was undiagnosed until I was about thirty-two years old. For many years, including much of my childhood, I suffered needlessly, and like so many others, I had no inkling about the real reason I had a "nervous stomach." Today, I laugh uproariously at the lactose-intolerance jokes that occasionally pop up on television programs and in popular movies. Even *Rolling Stone* magazine has had articles on the condition.

Knowing the tremendous benefit to be gained by sharing experiences with others, in 1987 I tried to develop the notion of a national support group by publishing the *Newsletter for People with Lactose Intolerance and Milk Allergy*. This unique publication offers the opportunity for readers across the country to share information, expert advice, special help for children, and milk-free recipes. The newsletter is still published today, six times a year, and information about subscribing to it can be found in the Appendix. One section of the newsletter is called "Readers' Forum" and features letters written to me by readers who ask questions about a milk-free diet or who offer their suggestions to other readers for good daily management ideas. It has become one of the most popular sections of the newsletter and for good reason: People feel great when they exchange ideas and concerns with one another about their individual circumstances.

So, in this book, I have decided to share with you some of the thousands of letters I have received over the years. These particular letters are from dairy-sensitive children and their parents. I hope that they will bring you some comfort and offer you some great advice for coping with your child and the milk-free lifestyle you are developing. Some of the letters will ask questions that I will answer; others will merely serve as a kind of emotional release for the family. All of the letters are real, but may have been edited somewhat for space. I hope you enjoy them. I want to express my gratitude to the newsletter readers who have written to me, who have taken me into their confidence and have furnished me with information, great recipes, and their terrific ideas for successful milk-free living.

Dear Jane,

My son and I are milk-sensitive. Since he turned ten months old, I have found no doctor willing to test him to discover if he is lactose intolerant (I don't think) or allergic (I think so). I have been lucky enough to discover that I am not a sufferer any longer of irritable bowel syndrome. My health problems have been solved by eliminating all dairy from my diet. This has been a delight, since I only did it at first to relieve my son's distress (he is breast-fed). Now I am angry that my doctor put me through a series of expensive tests years ago and attributed my health problems to "nerves." No one ever suggested I could have a sensitivity to milk! Thank you for the information on infants and children. I plan to make my parents read it so they can understand (and accept??!!) our food allergies.

    Very truly yours,
    Janet R.
    Haddon Heights, NJ

• • •

Dear Jane,

I recently saw a reference to your newsletter in the "Health" section of the Baltimore Sun. I would like more information as I have two children ages two and four who are allergic to cow's milk (not lactose intolerant). I also have some questions that I would appreciate an answer to, if you could help me. My children seem to be allergic to the casein factor of milk. Do you know if all ingredients with caseinate (i.e. sodium caseinate, potassium caseinate, etc.) as part of their name are derived from milk casein? Is there any other source of casein? If so, are different caseins cross-reactive? (My husband is an allergist, and he doesn't know the answers.) I would greatly appreciate whatever information you can give me. Thank you very much for your help.

    Sincerely,
    Gloria G.
    Columbia, MD

Dear Mrs. G.,

Yes, all items labeled caseinate contain a milk protein factor. Chemically they are a blend of casein and the other constituent, whether it is sodium, potassium, or calcium. Hope this helps.

• • •

Dear Jane,

My seven-year-old son has galactosemia and cannot have milk in any form. I am delighted to have discovered your newsletter. The recipes interest me most. Our biggest problem right now is finding interesting ways to fix a brown-bag lunch for school.

> *Terry F.*
> *Silvis, IL*

Dear Terry,

Check out Chapter 11 in this book!

• • •

Dear Jane,

Thank you for a very informative newsletter. We have a three-year-old who is very allergic to all dairy products. Thank goodness I started nursing her on day one. On the RAST she tests over 6000 percent (anything over 1000 percent is high), therefore she doesn't tolerate beef either. But, we've discovered buffalo which agrees with her and she loves it. And it is very lean and tasty. So, I've learned how to make changes and read all labels. Whey, too, is another form of milk. If she has just a morsel, this leads to a bad allergic reaction and asthma requiring Epipen Jr. [epinephrine]. This is why the [information regarding] the government experiment of preservatives of milk protein for fruits and vegetables is so disturbing. What will we do if this is done? Don't they realize the number of people who have milk allergies? Special treats she can have are Ice Bean, Tofutti, or Rice Dream, all made of frozen soy or tofu.

> *Thanks again!*
> *Kelly Z.*
> *Waverly, IA*

• • •

Dear Jane,

I am attempting to eliminate all milk and milk products from my daughter's diet. I have been buying bread which contains stearoyl lactylates. Are these milk derived? Do you have any bread recommendations? Thank you.

> *Sincerely,*
> *Pat B.*
> *Snellville, GA*

Dear Pat,

Stearoyl lactylate is a calcium derivative. It is not milk. Look for breads which are naturally milk-free such as "ethnic" breads including pita, French, Italian, and bagels.

• • •

Dear Jane,

I am sixteen years old and was born with galactosemia. It has been very difficult for me to find dairy substitutes. I recently heard about a product called Dairy Ease. I called their information number to see if this product would also work for people like me, but no one could answer this question. Can you tell me if people with galactosemia can use Dairy Ease and then eat real dairy products? Also, in your last newsletter someone asked if lactose intolerance applies to other foods than dairy products and the answer was no! But, [when I was] an infant my parents were told I could not have legumes [peas and beans], beets, liver, and sweetbreads. Were my parents misinformed or is this true for galactosemia?

> *Sincerely,*
> *Jodi S.*
> *Canadensis, PA*

Dear Jodi,

As a person with galactosemia, you cannot hydrolyze the monosaccharide galactose, which is found in lactose and is also a constituent of the digestion of legumes and beets and the other foods your parents were told you must avoid. Lactose is a disaccharide, that is, a double sugar composed of glucose and galactose, which must be hydrolyzed by the enzyme lactase. As a person with galactosemia, you cannot have galactose or lactose, because you do not have the proper enzymes for digesting either sugar. But people with lactose intolerance must only watch out for lactose, the sugar found in dairy foods, and may therefore eat legumes and beats, sweetbreads, etc. The product Dairy Ease is a lactase enzyme supplement, which will help hydrolyze the lactose by about 70 percent. That means there will still be 30 percent lactose remaining. I doubt that would be advisable for you. Better check with your doctor.

• • •

Dear Jane,

I have a two-and-a-half-year old son who is extremely milk allergic. We have received the first issue of your newsletter and are thankful and impressed. I would love to communicate with other parents with milk-allergic children and find out how they have coped. We have been told that our son should not attend the various multigroup children's activities (such as nursery school, etc.), and my son is such a social little boy, I'd hate to deprive him of the social stimulation.

Yours,
Sandy G.
Durham, NC

• • •

Dear Jane,

I am the mother of a thirteen-month-old child who is deathly allergic to milk and all other dairy products. His reaction to milk and anything with casein is frightening. He has severe respiratory reactions needing an Epipen Jr. injection and further hospital treatment. Needless to say, our lives have changed drastically. We have two other children ages six and three who have never had allergies to anything. My husband and I had and still have many questions. We see a doctor at St. Elizabeth's Hospital in Boston and he is super! We live with great fear that our son at age thirteen months will pick up something, somewhere, somehow, and well, I can't even think of it. I'm hoping to read how others cope with this allergy in this "milk, casein, lactalbumin, whey" world!

Thanks for listening,
Marci L.
Boston, MA

• • •

Dear Jane,

I have been disappointed in your recipe book because you listed so many recipes that contain chocolate. Chocolate has milk and caffeine in it, does it not? According to our doctor, these ingredients are in chocolate. Because of this, our daughter and I could not understand why chocolate was used in some of your recipes. Perhaps we both missed something or are not aware of something you know. Please let me hear from you concerning this as my daughter, granddaughter, and mother are all allergic to the milk products.

Sincerely,
Phyllis E.
Port Byron, IL

Dear Phyllis,

Not all chocolate contains milk! Cocoa powder and most baking chocolate are completely milk-free. Also there are several chocolate syrups and semisweet candies including chocolate morsels that contain no milk protein or lactose. Remember that milk fat is not milk protein or milk sugar. Please read the ingredient labels carefully and learn how to enjoy chocolate. A complete discussion of chocolate is found in this book in Chapter 2.

• • •

Dear Jane,

After lots of research I've come across your name as a resource for more information on lactose intolerance. We have an almost-three-year-old boy with a severe lactose intolerance. He's not growing like other siblings and the doctor we see does not believe his lactose intolerance is a problem. He just tells us to avoid dairy products. I give Conor Tums (two per day), Total cereal, a vitamin with iron and calcium, and orange juice with calcium to replace other foods rich in calcium. (He also eats broccoli.) Do you have any other suggestions?

Thank you in advance,
Chris M.
Reston, VA

Dear Chris,

Sounds like you are doing great with Conor. I'm always impressed with a three-year-old who eats broccoli.

• • •

Dear Jane,

My son has lactose intolerance and suffered with it for many years before we figured it out. We had done lots of "doctoring" including X-rays, sonograms, change of medications prescribed for his epilepsy, and so on. He's also severely mentally retarded and could not vocally express the problem which was part of his daily life. Instead he expressed his pain and discomfort as a behavior problem—and it baffled us for years, including many physicians, social workers, instructors, and family members. We now use Coffee Rich as a milk substitute and find Lactaid milk very digestible and an iced product called Tofulite a good substitute for ice cream. The Lactaid tablets are given to him several times a day during mealtimes. My son also takes prescribed medications which contain lactose. When giving my son the prescribed medication which does contain lactose, but is a medication that he must have, we also give him a Lactaid tablet with it. This also has proven to be effective.

Sincerely,
Barbara L.
Damariscotta, ME

• • •

Dear Jane,

My son has milk allergy. He has been advised to drink Tofu White in place of milk. It contains sodium caseinate. He has also been told he could eat Pizzasoy, which has casein in it. Neither of these products are a problem for him. Our biggest problem now is to find egg substitutes, but most things baked become crumbly. Any suggestions? The RAST test states he is extremely allergic to egg whites. Does this mean I could mix the yolks with egg replacer?

Thanks,
Donna V.
Iowa City, IA

Dear Donna,

Apparently, the products you mention do not contain enough casein to affect your son's allergic threshold. However, I would watch the egg replacements, most of them *are* egg whites! For baking, try applesauce instead of egg, or two tablespoons of apricot baby food per egg. You also might need to increase the oil in the recipe by a couple of teaspoons in order to make up for the fat lost by not including an egg yolk.

• • •

Dear Jane,

I thought maybe I could give some birthday party hints. Duncan Hines white cake mix is milk-free. I keep frozen cupcakes in the nurse's freezer at school for my daughter so she can still celebrate birthdays and I keep them frozen at home to take along to any parties we might get invited to. I take a little container of Mocha Mix Frozen Dessert for her ice cream and she parties along with everyone else.

> *Sincerely,*
> *Pat G.*
> *Phoenix, AZ*

• • •

Dear Jane,

My firstborn was diagnosed as being milk intolerant or having allergies to all dairy products. I've been having a very difficult time, she is only fifteen months old, and I don't seem to be doing a good job of knowing what to feed her. First, they put her back on Isomil formula (soybean). Well, how long will she use this product and how can I go about finding out how long she may be milk intolerant?? Second, I'm having difficulties feeding her; everything seems to contain milk, cheese, and dairy products. I'm becoming frustrated because on top of the allergy she is a fussy and picky eater. For all I know she may be allergic to other foods. Please help me with ideas for feeding a fifteen-month-old. Third, how old do people need to be to use the new products that allow milk-intolerant people to eat dairy products? Please help! I feel like I can't get answers to my questions and my fifteen-month-old can't express her feelings! Any help in dealing with this the best way possible would be greatly appreciated!

P.S. Can't thank you enough for finding the newsletter and support of people with milk intolerance!

Sincerely,

Sharon S.

Willkes-Barre, PA

Dear Sharon,

Your child was probably put back on infant formula in order to give her adequate nutrients and calories, which she was apparently not receiving without it. She can continue to use the formula well into her childhood in varying amounts if necessary to boost her nutrition. You need to ask your child's pediatrician to define her condition more carefully for you. You need to know whether she is allergic to milk or intolerant to lactose, or both. Then, you will be able to choose her foods more wisely. Also, books like this one and others will help you feed her dairy-free foods. After trying a variety of foods, you are bound to find some things she will enjoy. Don't give up! Write back if you need more help.

● ● ●

Dear Jane,

We recently visited Drake University in Des Moines, IA, and found it difficult to eat the college menu. Everything was covered in cheese or included dairy. Is it possible to live in Iowa?!! My son is lactose intolerant and is concerned about eating at the university he plans to go to. Any suggestions would be greatly appreciated.

Thank you,

Jeanette A.

Cherry Hill, NJ

Dear Jeanette,

Please plan to meet with the director of food services at your son's college. You should be able to receive a list of menus on a weekly or monthly basis which could help your son choose appropriate foods. Perhaps the food service director could work closely with your son as well. If not, make sure your son has access to a refrigerator or stove or microwave in order to prepare some of his own dairy-free meals or snacks. Lots of college kids live on pasta and vegetables or fresh fruit. You might also want to make sure he takes a multivitamin and/or calcium supplement, if you think he won't be getting enough nutrients from his diet. He may also require additional funds for eating in restaurants more often than usual. Good luck.

• • •

Dear Jane,

I can't wait to see your new book Raising Your Child Without Milk. Please offer it through the newsletter. I've always thought your logo (we call it anti-cow here) was so cute. Have you considered making her into a sticker? It'd be an easy way for me to label non-milk items for my three-year-old and for those who may baby-sit for me. She already knows the symbol from just being curious. It's just a thought!
  Sincerely,
  Donna D.
  Toms River, NJ

Dear Donna,

Thanks for the great idea. The neon red stickers proclaiming "Feed Me Dairy-Free" are now available. Also a T-shirt is being designed with the same logo for kids and adults. See the Appendix for more information!

• • •

Dear Jane,

I am writing in reference to any information you can provide me regarding hereditary fructose intolerance. Our eight-month-old son was recently diagnosed with this condition. I would be very appreciative of any information you might have available. Thank you very much for your time.
  Sincerely,
  Jann G.
  Seminole, FL

Dear Jann,

As you know, fructose intolerance is the inability to digest fructose, the simple sugar found in many fruits and some vegetables.

I have enclosed an article on fructose intolerance, which I wrote a few years ago. This should help you greatly. Fructose intolerance is a tough one to have because this sugar is so readily available in thousands of foods and other food products such as corn syrup. You will need some careful guidance from your child's pediatrician or a registered dietitian.

● ● ●

Dear Jane,

My daughter is five years old and has lactose intolerance. She has been lactose intolerant from birth on. I tried making my own macaroni and cheese. I used a basic macaroni and cheese recipe with your Basic White Sauce II (from the Dairy-Free Cookbook). The white sauce recipe was great. It was the cheese that didn't work. The cheese was creamy from the beginning but after it sat awhile the cheese was sticky and separated from the noodles. The cheese was Formagge Shredded Cheddar made by Galaxy Foods. I am hoping someone can come up with macaroni and cheese. Kids love macaroni and cheese!

Thank you,
Gail E.
Macedonia, OH

Dear Gail,

As you have discovered, the soy cheeses or lactose-reduced cheeses don't work the same way in recipes as regular dairy cheese. Some of them melt a little bit, only to ball up later, and others don't melt at all. I will try to work on a macaroni and "cheese" recipe, but might not have any luck. You could give your daughter the macaroni with milk-free margarine and skip the "cheese" part, although I know it isn't quite the same. Or, you might prepare a "creamed" noodle casserole using the Basic White Sauce Recipe and adding tuna or chicken chunks and vegetables and topping it with crumbled corn flakes or potato chips for extra flavor. It might satisfy your daughter's desire for a creamy, textured noodley dish.

● ● ●

Dear Jane,

I've been receiving your newsletter for several years now and find it very helpful. I was hoping you could help me with a big problem I have. My six-year-old daughter is lactose intolerant, gluten intolerant, and allergic to soy and corn. I do not find that manufacturers are totally honest when it comes to ingredient labeling. The new law may help with fat percentages, etc., but not with ingredients. I will purchase a product that doesn't include corn syrup on their label and when I call the manufacturer to verify that there are none of my child's allergens in it, I find out that the fruit concentrate is enhanced with corn grain or a seltzer fruit juice has no sugar, but it does have caramel color which is from corn syrup. Help please? How can I determine what products contain what ingredients? My method is very time-consuming and costly.

   Thank you very much,
   Lisa L.
   Port Jefferson Station, Long Island, NY

Dear Lisa,

You have a difficult problem, indeed. All ingredients are not necessarily on food labels, because they may be constituents of other ingredients, such as the caramel/corn syrup connection you mention. Your learning about food ingredients and knowing that caramel coloring is derived from corn syrup will be invaluable. It is true that you will have to maintain a vigilance over manufactured foods which you give to your daughter, and you are to be commended for trying so hard to hunt for allergens that bother her. It may be impossible, however, to always protect her from allergens. In that case, you may have to rely more on fresh foods, which you can prepare at home and are free of manufactured food allergens. Fresh meats, fish, poultry, fruits, and vegetables will need to be the staples of your child's diet. Also search out health-food stores and other whole-food outlets for specially made "manufactured" foods that are corn or wheat or soy free. Check the appendix of this book for more help.

• • •

Dear Jane,

My eight-year-old daughter is very allergic to milk products. Eating out is always a challenge, but we have developed a sort of repertoire of "safe" meals. One of these is tuna-fish salad, which she loves. Recently she reacted to the tuna fish served at a Florida restaurant (her reaction progressed to head-to-toe hives and breathing difficulties) although I had specifically asked whether the tuna-fish salad included any dairy products such as cheese and was told it was just basic tuna-fish salad—tuna and mayonnaise. Several days later I went back and again asked about ingredients—they had used sour cream in with their tuna salad! This reminded me so much of the case of the Rhode Island college student who died from an anaphylactic reaction to the secret ingredient of peanut butter in chili, that I had to ask you to pass along the warning. Tuna-fish salad might be made with sour cream mixed in it. Luckily for us we were able to medicate my daughter in time.

Sincerely,
Anne M.
Princeton, NJ

• • •

Dear Jane,

My grandson has recently been diagnosed as having a severe lactose intolerance. I have been involved in calling different places—grocery stores and restaurants and bakeries—as to the different foods that are parve—lactose-free! I also heard that the Ambrosia Chocolate Factory makes a parve chocolate, but after talking to a few employees of the company, I am skeptical! I would like to know who checks up on parve products. Does the government do any investigating for this?

Thank you,
Mrs. Kerwin B.
Greendale, WI

Dear Mrs. B.,

No, the government does not police manufacturers who print the word "Parve" on their labels.

• • •

Dear Jane,

Hi! I need some help, information, or anything that will help my baby and myself to cope with this problem. For me it's rather devastating— dairy is my favorite food group (ice cream, milk, cheeses, yogurts, cream sauces, cheese cake, etc. . . .). Now my mouth salivates, but the rest of me is a medical mess. My baby has no dairy products and she won't take her soy formula any longer. I don't want to see her in that kind of pain without being able to tell me if it is a tummy ache or what. She's fourteen months old. Any pointers or tips would be helpful.

> *Thank you so much,*
> *Solange G.*
> *Portland, OR*

Dear Solange,

It sounds like you need some help from your child's pediatrician, who should be able to offer your daughter a dairy-free, soy-free infant formula alternative. You are also going to have to learn to like other foods—both of you—and believe me, there are lots of appetizing and tasty foods other than dairy. Besides, did you ever stop to think of how much saturated fat and cholesterol you are eating when you eat so much dairy? Your heart and arteries will appreciate your cutting back.

● ● ●

Dear Jane,

I hope you receive this—my fingers are crossed. I just finished reading your Dairy-Free Cookbook. The information answered so many questions the doctors have not been able to answer for ten years! Thank you! My son and I are still grinning after trying your Basic Vanilla Ice Cream. . . . It's been a hard summer for this ice-cream-loving ten-year-old! We will continue to experiment with your recipes, but this mom needs to learn more to expand on our diet limitations. We are both allergic to protein found in dairy products.

> *Many thanks!*
> *Peggy and Kevin B.*
> *Long Lake, MN*

● ● ●

Dear Jane,

I recently purchased two products because they were labeled lactose-free. When I read the small print I found that the main ingredient in each is whey. Now I am afraid to serve them to my family. Also, I would like to warn your readers to be careful of all bread products. Many multigrain or ethnic breads and dinner rolls contain whey. I have had problems with English muffins, raisin breads, stuffing mixes, bread crumbs, or any food breaded with crumbs. Not even soups or ramen noodles can be considered safe. One of the new "healthy" soups on the market has whey in the chicken noodle variety. Shoppers should check their holiday turkeys to be sure they have not been injected with a lactose solution!

Sincerely,
Michele B.
Eastlake, OH

Dear Michele,
Thanks for the tips. You make a good case for cooking at home. As you have seen, whey is in so many, many products. That's because the cheese industry in this country is huge—Americans are eating more cheese than ever before. One of the by-products of cheese production is whey, which is now being sold off to food manufacturers and tossed into just about everything it seems!

• • •

Dear Jane,

I was very excited to hear that you have produced a newsletter for people who are lactose intolerant. This is a condition I have had to deal with personally for most of my life along with having children also with this condition. I am interested in knowing if you have addressed the problem of medication. I do know lactose is used as a filler in many medications. I have personally wanted to get pharmaceutical firms to stop using lactose, but I realize that I'm only one person. Through the use of your newsletter, many people can lobby together and in numbers we can perhaps effect change.

Sincerely,
Linda R.
Rochester, NY

• • •

Dear Jane,

My daughter, Amanda, cannot digest any milk, cheese, milk chocolate, or anything like that without getting extremely bad diarrhea. She is fifteen years old and is five foot four inches tall and weighs 101 pounds. She is very active and is on her high-school basketball team. We tried taking the lactose pills, but they do not help at all. At first they did, but she cannot use them now. We took her to her doctor and all she said was "that it is just something she has to live with." I have a friend who is a doctor and he suggests going to Vanderbilt to the Children's Gastrology Dept. What I want to know is, is there anything you can suggest that we try, or do you think it should be checked out further?

> *Sincerely,*
> *Mary H.*
> *Baxter, TN*

Dear Mary,

If your daughter is lactose intolerant, but otherwise healthy, there probably is no need for further testing. What you will need to do is learn how to provide her with a healthful dairy-free diet. Because she is so active, she will require lots of calories per day, perhaps between 2,200 and 3,000 or more. She may also require a calcium supplement to protect her bones against osteoporosis later in life, although the basketball and working-out she undoubtedly does in training are helping her muscles become strong and her bones become dense. It might not be a bad idea to consult with a registered dietitian who can assess your daughter's physical needs and recommend a specific dairy-free, high-calorie diet.

• • •

Dear Jane,

I love your newsletter! It was such a relief to finally hear some information on milk allergy. My infant son has a severe case. When he was five weeks old he started bleeding rectally (about 1/4 cup each time) and started losing weight. Finally at nine weeks he was diagnosed with milk-

protein intolerance. He had developed small bleeding ulcers in the lower intestine. He was put on Pregestimil formula and has done great. He is now eight months old and we are trying to educate ourselves on milk-free diets.

Thank you,
Amanda G.
Murrieta, CA

• • •

Dear Jane,

My son is four years old and has never had a sip of milk. On his first birthday he was given one teaspoon of ice cream, which resulted in red itchy eyes and lines. His pediatrician has said he should be able to drink milk when he gets older since both my husband and I have no allergy to milk or dairy products. I do not know if my son is lactose intolerant or has a milk allergy to the protein in cow's milk I have read about. I feel he should be sent to an allergist for evaluation. The pediatrician has said there is nothing they can do, but I've been in the dark about this for four years now.

I've given my son some foods which contain whey and casein which he seems to tolerate. However, sometimes he will tell me his mouth hurts after eating some things and I can't figure out what is happening to him. Once I gave him a half a slice of cheese, which he ate, but then two hours later he vomited. I feel I need some real help on what to do. He still drinks ProSobee formula. Is there any other milk substitute he can drink? I've read about Vitamite, but do I give this to my son when I do not know if he is milk allergic or intolerant to lactose?

A very confused and concerned parent,
Debra D.
Morton, PA

Dear Debra,

Please understand the hallmark difference between lactose intolerance and milk allergy. The first condition elicits digestive distress symptoms such as bloating, gas, and diarrhea. The second (milk allergy) causes typically allergic responses in the sensitive person. These include many of the symptoms you describe when talking about your son: red eyes, itching, vomiting, discomfort about the lips.

If I were to guess, I would say that he has an allergy to milk protein. That you were able to give him some whey and casein may indicate that his tolerance level could handle the amount ingested. And, it is true that his tolerance level for milk protein will increase with age. As for testing, your pediatrician makes a good point for not testing your child for food allergies, because at this age allergy testing is generally not reliable for food.

However, that does not mean there is nothing you can do. A consultation with a pediatric allergist could be very beneficial for you and your son. He may be allergic to other substances, which the allergist could determine, and perhaps the allergist could give you better information regarding your son's allergies in general. Vitamite, while it contains no lactose, does contain milk proteins and may not be suitable for your child.

• • •

Dear Jane,

I recently read an article about you in a newspaper from Washington, Pennsylvania. I am fifteen years old and have a spastic colon (an intestinal problem) which has restricted me to a diet of no lactose, low sugar, and low-fat meals. I would greatly appreciate a copy of your milk-free recipes as I am sure it would add a greater variety to my diet. Thank you very much for your time and for helping make eating for people like me a lot more enjoyable.

Sincerely,
Mindy P.
Pittsburgh, PA

• • •

Dear Jane,

A friend of mine told me about you. My twelve-year-old son has been off milk for two years now. He was just retested for milk allergy and it turned out negative, but milk still seems to upset his stomach. He also has irritable bowel syndrome. I was wondering if your newsletter would help us.

Yours truly,
Doreen S.
Omaha, NE

Dear Doreen,

It seems as though your son's allergy test is not a true reflection of his condition. Perhaps he gets sick to his stomach after drinking milk because he is in fact intolerant to the lactose in milk, but no longer allergic to the milk protein. Also, with a diagnosis of IBS, he may need more careful treatment. About 60 percent of people diagnosed with IBS are, in fact, lactose intolerant. I would recommend that you take your son to see a pediatric gastroenterologist, who may be better able to help you sort out his digestive problems and could test the boy for lactose intolerance. In the meantime, I wouldn't give him any milk if it makes him sick. Digestive distress and diarrhea will surely exacerbate an irritable bowel.

• • •

Dear Jane,

My daughter, Jaime, who is eight years old, has been diagnosed as lactose intolerant. She was hospitalized for Shigella and this caused the damage and left her lactose intolerant. I have found your cookbooks, to say the least, to be a godsend! Trying to get an eight-year-old to accept that she cannot eat certain foods without making her feel too "different" has been a challenge. I know this holiday season will be very difficult for Jaime, this being her first year as "intolerant" and having several relatives who do not understand about her dietary restrictions (even though they have been told). Any advice you can give me would be greatly appreciated!

Thank you,
Connie G.
Lorain, OH

Dear Connie,

Just in time for Jaime is the book *Milk-Free Holiday Cooking*, a collection of dairy-free family recipes shared by newsletter readers. I hope you enjoy it. Maybe you should get several copies for the relatives.

• • •

Dear Jane,

Your cookbook has been invaluable to me ever since my six-year-old (whose favorite foods were milk and bagels) was diagnosed as being lactose intolerant in June. I became lactose intolerant several years ago, but it's a whole different ball game when a six-year-old suddenly can't have the very things she loves.

    Sincerely,
    Julie C.
    Louisville, KY

• • •

Dear Jane,

I just read an article in our area newspaper about food allergies. My son has some food allergies that we know about, milk allergy and bananas. He is now nine years old, but we have been dealing with his milk allergy since he was four years old. He has a lot of allergies to things such as grass, trees, molds, dust, weeds, and also animals and so on. I won't bore you with the long list. He also has asthma. I was surprised to see products on the market for people allergic to milk and other allergies. I didn't know I could get yogurt made with soy. It's called Soyalatte and Tofutti frozen dessert.

    Sincerely,
    Sharon H.
    Columbus, OH

• • •

Dear Jane,

My grandson has had distressing symptoms from the time he was born, and my daughter, who was nursing him, discovered by process of elimination that if she ate no milk products, he was fine. He is two now, and can eat Dannon Plain Yogurt with no problem, although other brands, which seem to have more ingredients, cause him trouble. He is also allergic to egg whites. Probably none of this is new to you, but I thought it might be of some interest.

    Yours truly,
    Patricia D.
    Baton Rouge, LA

• • •

Dear Jane,

Our son, Adam, age five, had all the problems of milk intolerance: coughing through the night, vomiting frequently, upset stomach, and a general weak and tired existence. We were literally poisoning our son's system with dairy products. Milk and cheese were eaten just about every day in some form. We took him to an allergist who threw some very technical terms at us, but didn't help very much.

Then we discovered a holistic physician who zeroed in on the dairy products and wheat products and sugar, which are just about in every product consumed today. Whether it be sorbitol, corn syrup, or just plain sugar. Needless to say, breakfast, which consisted of cereal with milk, was nothing but sugar and lactose and casein. What a terrible way for my son to start each day! Since we have discovered this problem a year ago, our son Adam is now a happy, well-adjusted child.

Sincerely,
Bob and Deb D.
Ocean Bluff, MA

• • •

Dear Jane,

I am eleven years old and have been lactose intolerant for only about a year. I have tried calcium-rich orange juice and Tums, which have extra calcium, to get the calcium my body needs, but the orange juice gave me stomach aches, and the Tums were extremely sweet and kind of disgusting, although some people might want to use them as an extra source of calcium. Right now I am trying to eat more vegetables like spinach and broccoli. I love this newsletter!

Sincerely,
Rose L.
Montpelier, VT

Dear Rose,

Congratulations on your trying to find alternative sources of calcium. It shows how well you understand the importance of calcium in your diet, and how much you respect yourself and your body. Here are a few other suggestions: You might want to take a calcium supplement that you do *not* chew, but rather swallow, or drink some of the new calcium-fortified apple and other juice products like Gerber's Graduates (we won't tell). You might also want to eat calcium-fortified breads like those now being produced by Wonder. Have you tried tofu? If you whip it in the blender with some onion soup mix, you have a nice dip for vegetables, maybe even that broccoli you are trying to eat more often.

• • •

Dear Jane,

I have subscribed to your newsletter for two and a half years after discovering that our child, who is now three and a half, has a severe milk allergy. Our child was diagnosed at seven weeks old. She showed signs of diarrhea with blood streaks as allergic reactions to the cow's milk I was drinking while she was being breast-fed. Allergists recommended avoidance of all dairy products. By one year of age, one spoonful of milk caused repeated vomiting and an outbreak of hives on her face and especially around her mouth. By age one and a half, we discovered that exposure to milk through skin contact produces hives. Needless to say, we are very concerned about her condition and need to continue to search for any answers. If there is any possibility to desensitize and achieve even the slightest improvement, I feel it would be best to start at this young age. My concern, however, is not to make an already severe milk allergy even worse.

Sincerely,
Connie L.
Columbus, OH

Dear Connie,

When you refer to desensitization, I assume you mean exposing your daughter to small amounts of milk on a regular basis in order for her body to stop reacting to the milk. But, no, I'm afraid that desensitization is not possible or advisable for children your daughter's age. I have seen no research or scientific studies that prove that desensitization will work; in fact, to the contrary, children with severe milk allergies run the risk of developing anaphylactic shock through exposure to milk proteins. Please discuss this matter with your daughter's pediatric allergist for a more complete answer to your question.

• • •

Dear Jane,

Our son has a severe milk/dairy allergy and has been admitted to the hospital many, many times because of it. The only way we've found to prevent these dangerous asthma attacks he experiences is to totally avoid dairy! All the doctors we speak to say this is a dangerous practice as he gets absolutely nothing from the dairy food group! We've had nine months asthma-free since excluding dairy totally from his diet—are we sitting on a time bomb nutritionally? He's been in excellent health, better than he's ever been. Is it safe to exclude the dairy group in its entirety? No, we don't give any vitamin supplements as we have had a dietitian give him a diet taking into consideration the calcium deficit. His diet is high in salmon with bones, sardines, broccoli, green vegetables, nuts, shrimp, plus he eats fish, poultry, pork, and all vegetables and fruits plus grains. We instate his diet and repeat foods every four days. He eats extremely well, never touches candy, chocolate, pop, cookies, etc. He just turned eight years old, weights fifty-two pounds, is fifty inches tall, very clever and accepts his allergies with respect and maturity. He is also allergic to antibiotics and several other foods, including eggs, peanuts, as well as cats, dogs, etc.

> *Thank you,*
> *Gail T. (concerned mother)*
> *Scottsdale, AZ*

Dear Gail,

What more could you ask for than a healthy child who eats all the foods that are good for him and avoids all the foods and other allergens that are bad for him? Congratulations on his and your accomplishments.

11

Feed Me—
Dairy-Free!

Here are some recipes for you to enjoy along with your children. None of the recipes contains milk in any form. They are all completely milk-protein-free and lactose-free. If your child can tolerate some dairy products, please feel free to add them as you wish. Also, you will notice that most of these recipes are not heavily seasoned. Again, you will have to adjust them to your own taste.

At the end of this chapter you will find suggestions for substitutions that will help you adapt your own family's favorite recipes to a milk-free diet. Remember that when a recipe calls for a milk substitute it means that you may use the substitute of your choice: This could be either infant formula, soy milk, orange juice, nondairy creamer, lactose-reduced milk, applesauce, or something else—whatever you feel is appropriate for your child and for the recipe (see Table 11.1). You may have to experiment a little to get things just right, but please don't give up too quickly. Perhaps if you include your child in the cooking process, you will both have some fun learning to prepare these special foods together.

The recipes are divided into classifications that are a little unusual, perhaps, because I do not subscribe to the notion that certain foods must be fed at certain times of the day. Therefore, you won't find recipes designated as suitable for breakfast or lunch or dinner. Rather, you will find recipes for main meals, fruits and veggies, snacks, treats, brown-bagging, and birthday party ideas. Feel free to serve soup for breakfast, veggies and dip for lunch, and scrambled eggs for dinner. More important than what your child eats when, is what your child eats, period.

Table 11.1 Substitutions

WHEN RECIPE CALLS FOR:	SUBSTITUTE:
1 cup milk	$1/2$ cup nondairy creamer blended with $1/2$ cup water
	$1/2$ cup juice blended with $1/2$ cup water
	1 cup water or juice
	1 cup soy milk
	1 cup infant formula
	For baking: 1 cup water + 2 tablespoons milk-free margarine
	For yeast dough: 1 cup ginger ale
1 cup buttermilk	$1/2$ cup nondairy creamer + $1/2$ cup water + 1 tablespoon vinegar or lemon juice
1 cup sour milk	Same as above
Light cream	Nondairy creamer or soy milk
Heavy cream	Milk-free whipping cream or meringue
Sour cream	Mayonnaise + 1 tablespoon sugar
Cream cheese	Mayonnaise

Remember, too, that dairy-sensitive children come in all sizes from 12 pounds to 120 pounds, so not all of these recipes will be appropriate for your child's age. Some recipes will definitely be more suitable for a four-year-old than a fourteen-year-old, and some recipes will only be appropriate for older children, rather than toddlers. Please make your choices according to your child's needs.

I would like to take this opportunity to thank the many readers of my newsletter who have so graciously shared their recipes with me and have allowed me, in turn, to share them with you. I also want to thank my mother, Lama Shetzer, and my friends Dale Frankel and Mary Jo Fitzpatrick for their delicious contributions to this recipe section. I hope your family enjoys these nutritious milk-free recipes, and that they bring some welcome variety into your child's dairy-free lifestyle.

Main Meals

Egg in a Hole

1 piece soft bread
Milk-free margarine
1 egg

Using a glass (or a cookie cutter) about the same diameter as the slice of bread, cut out a circle of bread. In a small frying pan, melt about 2 teaspoons milk-free margarine (use less in a non-stick frying pan). Place both the circle and the ring of bread in the frying pan. Break an egg into the center of the ring of bread. Cook over medium heat until browned on the bottom. With a wide spatula, turn over the bread circle and the egg in the hole to brown for just a few moments. Remove and serve.

YIELD: 1 serving

Red Eyes (Deviled Salmon Eggs)

4 eggs
1 small can red salmon with bones
1 tablespoon sweet pickle relish
1 teaspoon Worcestershire sauce
Mayonnaise

Place eggs in a pot with enough water to cover the eggs. Cook until the water reaches a rolling boil. Turn off heat, remove pot, cover, and set aside for 15 minutes. Drain salmon. In a small bowl, mash salmon with the bones until well blended. Add relish, and Worcestershire sauce, and blend well. Set aside. Run hard-boiled eggs under cold water to cool. Remove shells and discard. Cut each egg in half. Remove yolks and add them to the salmon mixture. Blend yolks into salmon mixture, adding enough mayonnaise to reach desired consistency. Fill the egg white centers with salmon mixture. Refrigerate for at least 30 minutes to allow the flavors to blend.

YIELD: 2–4 servings

Green Soup and Ham

3 tablespoons milk-free margarine
2 pounds leeks, split, washed, and chopped
    (onions may be used)
2 carrots, peeled, chopped
2 celery stalks, chopped
3 cloves garlic, chopped
12–14 cups water
1 pound green split peas
2 teaspoons salt
1 teaspoon freshly ground black pepper
1 cup cooked broccoli, pureed
2 cups diced cooked ham

In a large soup pot, melt 3 tablespoons milk-free margarine. Add leeks, carrots, celery, and garlic. Over medium heat, sauté vegetables until soft but not browned, about 5 minutes. Add 10 cups of water, the split peas, the salt, and the pepper. Cook, stirring occasionally, 45 minutes. Add 2 cups more water. Cook 30 minutes longer or until the peas are very soft and fall apart, adding water as necessary. Remove and cool. In a blender or food processor, puree 3 cups soup. Add back to the soup pot along with the pureed broccoli and diced ham. Blend gently and warm through.

YIELD: 12–14 servings

Fiesta Scramble

6 eggs
1/4 cup orange juice
Milk-free margarine
1 large jar prepared salsa
6 soft flour tortillas

Beat eggs slightly. Add orange juice and beat again until frothy. Scramble eggs in melted margarine until loosely cooked. While the eggs are cooking, warm the salsa in a saucepan. Scoop a serving of eggs on each tortilla. Roll up and place in a baking pan. Top with warm salsa and serve.

YIELD: 6 servings

Corn Chowder

4 medium potatoes, peeled and diced
1 medium onion, chopped
2 stalks celery, chopped
2 cups chicken broth
1 (10-ounce) package frozen whole kernel corn
2 tablespoons milk-free margarine
2 tablespoons flour
1 cup milk substitute (do not use juice)
Salt and pepper

In a medium saucepan, combine potatoes, onion, celery, and broth. Bring to a boil. Cover, reduce heat, and simmer for 20 minutes or until potatoes are tender. Add corn and continue to simmer for 7 to 8 minutes. Set aside 1 cup of this mixture to cool to room temperature. When it is ready, puree it in a blender. Return this mixture to the saucepan. In a small saucepan, melt margarine over low heat, stir in flour, and cook for about 1 minute, stirring constantly. Slowly add milk substitute and cook until the sauce is thick and smooth. Add to corn chowder mixture. Season to taste with salt and pepper.

Note: Try adding some cubed tofu to this recipe for extra calcium and protein.

YIELD: 4–6 servings

Cool Kasha Salad

2 cups white raisins
3 cups cooked barley
3 cups cooked kasha (use chicken broth or bouillon as the liquid)
2 ounces slivered almonds
$1/4$ cup chopped green onion
2 teaspoons salt
$1/2$ cup olive oil
$1/4$ cup white cider vinegar
2 teaspoons sugar

Soak raisins in warm water to cover until they are plump. Prepare barley and kasha. Drain raisins. Blend all ingredients in a large serving bowl and refrigerate 2 to 3 hours to let flavors blend. Serve cold.

YIELD: 8 servings

Monterrey Chicken Spread

$1/4$ cup mayonnaise
$1/4$ cup prepared salsa
1 cup finely chopped cooked chicken (turkey may be used)
$1/2$ cup chopped toasted almonds
1 teaspoon chopped onion

In a small bowl, mix together mayonnaise and salsa. In another bowl, blend chicken, almonds, and onion. Add enough mayonnaise/salsa mix to moisten chicken to a good spreading consistency. Spread on flour tortillas or bread, or serve as a dip with corn chips.

YIELD: Serves 4

Cream of Carrot Soup

Vegetable oil
4 cups chopped carrots
1/4 cup uncooked rice
6 cups chicken broth
6 cups water
Salt and pepper to taste

In a large soup pot, pour only enough oil to cover the bottom.
Heat until very hot. Add carrots. Lower heat and cook until they
soften slightly. Add rice and cook for one minute, tossing gently.
Add broth and water and cook until rice and carrots are soft.
Add salt and pepper to taste. Let set until room temperature.
Puree in a blender until smooth. Serve hot or cold.

YIELD: 12 servings

Bruce's Favorite Lentil Soup

3/4 cup dried lentils (choose a pretty color!)
1 cup chopped onion
2 cloves garlic, minced
1 1/2 cups shredded carrots
3 pieces of celery, chopped
2 tablespoons chopped fresh parsley
4 cups chicken broth
3 cups water
2 bay leaves
1/2 teaspoon cumin
Pinch of thyme
Pinch of turmeric or curry powder
Salt and pepper to taste
2 tablespoons lemon juice
1 cup cubed cooked chicken (optional)
Fresh dill

In a large soup pot combine lentils, onion, garlic, carrots, celery, parsley, chicken broth, water, bay leaves, cumin, thyme, turmeric, salt and pepper. Cover and simmer for 50 to 60 minutes or until lentils are tender. Remove bay leaves. Stir in the lemon juice and chicken and heat through. Adjust the seasonings as desired.

YIELD: Serves 4–6

Mildest Chili con Carne

1 pound chopped beef
1 pound ground turkey
$1/4$ cup milk-free margarine
1 medium onion, diced
1 stalk celery, diced
1 green pepper, diced
1 (28-ounce) can peeled whole tomatoes
1 (15-ounce) can pinto beans
1 (16-ounce) can red kidney beans
2 teaspoons chili powder
1 teaspoon paprika
1 teaspoon salt
$1/2$ teaspoon pepper

In a frying pan, brown beef and turkey. Remove and drain. Set aside. In a large saucepan, melt margarine. Sauté onion, celery, and green pepper until soft. Add tomatoes. Blend vegetables and bring to a boil. Add meats. Cover and simmer 10 minutes. Add beans and spices. Simmer 30 to 45 minutes.

YIELD: 8–10 servings.

One, Two, Three, Shells!

1 (12-ounce) box jumbo pasta shells
1 1/2 pounds ground beef (or beef combined with turkey or
    sausage)
1 (30-ounce) jar milk-free spaghetti sauce (homemade is great!)
1 cup broccoli florets, chopped
Nonstick cooking spray

Prepare pasta shells according to manufacturer's directions, but
cook only until pliable, not all the way through. Rinse in cold
water and set aside. In a frying pan, brown beef. Remove and
drain. Spray a 9-by-13-inch glass baking dish with nonstick cooking spray. Spread a few tablespoons of spaghetti sauce on the bottom of the baking dish. In a bowl, combine beef, broccoli florets,
and remaining spaghetti sauce, reserving 1 cup. Fill each shell
with this mixture and place in the baking dish. Line the bottom
first, then start a second layer. Top with remaining sauce. Bake at
350° for about 30 minutes, or until pasta is tender.

YIELD: 8–10 servings

Dale's World-Famous Mushroom Barley Soup

1 cup sliced mushrooms
1 large diced onion
3 stalks celery, chopped
2 carrots, grated
1 cup barley (uncooked)
3 quarts water
1 teaspoon pepper
2 teaspoons salt
1 bay leaf

Blend all ingredients in a large soup pot. Cook on low heat about
2 hours. Add water, as necessary. Remove bay leaf before serving.

YIELD: 8–10 servings

MJ's Chicken in a Crockpot

2 carrots, sliced
2 onions, sliced
2 celery stalks with leaves, cut in 1-inch pieces
1 (3-pound) whole broiler/fryer chicken
2 teaspoons salt
$1/2$ teaspoon coarse black pepper
$1/2$ cup chicken broth
$1/2$ teaspoon basil

Place carrots, onions, and celery in bottom of crockpot. Add whole chicken (use a skinless chicken if you prefer to cut back on the fat). Top with salt, pepper, and broth. Sprinkle basil over the top. Cover and cook on low 8 to 10 hours. (High: Cook 4 to 5 hours using 1 cup broth.)

YIELD: 6–8 servings

Anything á la King

Make the following white sauce. Then add chunks of cooked fish, cooked chicken or turkey, and a variety of green and yellow vegetables. Serve over cooked noodles, rice, or toast.

2 tablespoons milk-free margarine
2 tablespoons flour
$1/2$ teaspoon salt
$1/4$ teaspoon white pepper
2 cups milk substitute (do not use juice) or chicken broth

Melt margarine in a small pan. Remove from heat. Add, flour, salt, and pepper. Return to low heat. Add liquid gradually, stirring constantly until thick.

YIELD: About 4 cups ($1/2$ cup per serving)

Cowboy Stew

1^1/$_2$ pounds stewing beef (veal or lamb may be used)
1 can tomato soup
1 package milk-free dry onion soup mix
1 can kidney beans
1 can beef broth
1 pound carrots, sliced into 3-inch chunks
8 small red potatoes, peeled

Place all ingredients into a 3-quart casserole. Bake, covered, in a 300° oven for 4 to 5 hours.

Yield: 8 servings

Chicken 'n' Brown Gravy

2 tablespoons flour
^{1}/$_8$ teaspoon dried thyme leaves
^{1}/$_4$ teaspoon salt
^{1}/$_8$ teaspoon pepper
^{1}/$_2$ teaspoon paprika
4 skinless, boneless chicken breasts
Olive oil

Blend flour with thyme, salt, pepper, and paprika. Coat chicken breasts with seasoned flour. Sauté in olive oil about 7 minutes on each side, or until cooked through. Remove and drain. Transfer to a deep serving dish and keep warm. Top with hot Brown Gravy.

Yield: 4 servings

Brown Gravy

2 tablespoons milk-free margarine
1 small onion, diced
2–3 tablespoons flour

2 cups beef broth
$1/2$ teaspoon brown gravy enhancer (Kitchen Bouquet,
    for example)

In the same pan that the chicken was cooked in, add margarine and melt. Brown diced onion and blend with the chicken bits and other remaining seasonings from the chicken. Add flour and blend until smooth. Slowly add beef broth and cook until mixture boils and thickens. Add brown gravy enhancer for color. Strain if necessary.

YIELD: 3 cups

California Lavash

On a whole round of soft lavash bread, spread dijon mustard evenly. Top with layers of thinly sliced turkey and ham. Next, add thin slices of avocado and a thick layer of sprouts. Sprinkle chopped green onion on top. Carefully roll up the lavash bread and wrap tightly in plastic wrap. Refrigerate for at least 1 hour. To serve, remove plastic wrap and slice the sandwich in 2-inch slices.

VARIATIONS

Middle Eastern Lavash   Spread the bread with hummus. Top with slices of cooked, peeled eggplant, sliced olives, and chopped tomato. Top with chopped fresh parsley and chopped green onion. Roll, refrigerate, and slice.

Down-Home Lavash   Spread the bread with ham salad. Top with cold cooked greens such as collards or kale. Sprinkle with chopped celery and onion. Roll, refrigerate, and slice.

High Calcium Lavash   Spread the bread with a combination of mashed canned salmon and canned shrimp that has been blended with mayonnaise and lemon juice. Top with crumbled tofu and chopped green onion. Roll, refrigerate, and slice.

Flapjacks with Molasses-Orange Maple Syrup

1 cup flour
1 tablespoon baking powder
1 tablespoon sugar
$1/2$ teaspoon salt
1 egg, well beaten
$1/2$ cup orange juice
$1/2$ cup water
2 tablespoons vegetable oil
Milk-free margarine for the griddle

In a deep bowl, mix together flour, baking powder, sugar, and salt. In a separate bowl, combine egg with juice, water, and oil. Add egg and liquids to dry ingredients, stirring just until moist. Let mixture rest for 30 seconds. Spoon or pour batter onto greased, hot griddle. Cook pancakes on the first side until bubbles appear on upper surface. Turn over and cook until bottom is golden. Top with syrup.

YIELD: 4 servings

MOLASSES-ORANGE MAPLE SYRUP

$1/4$ cup blackstrap molasses
1 teaspoon orange zest
$3/4$ cup maple syrup

In a small bowl, combine ingredients and mix well.

YIELD: 4 servings.

Kids' Chicken á l'Orange

2 chicken legs with thighs or breasts with wing pieces
Salt and pepper to taste
$1/2$ cup calcium-fortified orange juice
2 tablespoons milk-free margarine, melted

Place chicken in a small baking dish and season with salt and pepper. In a small bowl, blend melted margarine with orange juice and pour over chicken. Bake at 375° for about 45 minutes.

YIELD: 2 servings

Salmon Croquettes with Hollandaise Sauce

1 (15.5-ounce) can red salmon
1 egg, slightly beaten
$^1/_2$ cup chopped red onion
$^1/_2$ cup mashed potatoes
Salt and pepper to taste
Vegetable oil

Drain salmon. In a large bowl, mash salmon and bones well. Blend with egg, onion, mashed potatoes, salt, and pepper. Form into small patties and refrigerate for at least 30 minutes. Sauté in oil until well browned on both sides. Serve with Hollandaise Sauce.

YIELD: 6 servings

HOLLANDAISE SAUCE

3 egg yolks
2 tablespoons lemon juice
$^3/_2$ cup milk-free margarine

Beat egg yolks and lemon juice for 2 minutes with an electric mixer. Melt margarine in a saucepan and slowly pour hot margarine into egg mixture, beating at high speed until fluffy.

Note: Add peas or broccoli florets to sauce for added nutrition.

YIELD: 1 cup

Cheeseless Pizza

1 (16-ounce) prepared focaccia bread
Olive oil
2 cups mashed potatoes
Mushrooms, chopped
Green pepper, chopped
Olives, chopped
Pepperoni slices

Place the focaccia bread on an ungreased cookie sheet. Spread olive oil over the bread. Spread mashed potatoes over the oil. Use more or less, as desired. Top with chopped mushrooms, green pepper, olives, or whatever pizza toppings your child likes. Arrange pepperoni slices on top. Bake in a preheated 450° oven for about 20 minutes or until heated through and golden brown.

YIELD: 6 servings

Toddler Fish Dinner

1 fillet of sole
1 cup chicken broth
2 broccoli florets, steamed until soft
1 tablespoon baby rice cereal, mixed with infant formula or
    other milk substitute (do not use juice)

Rinse fish and pat dry. In a frying pan, bring chicken broth to a boil and set the fillet in the pan. Bring to a second boil, reduce heat, cover and simmer until fish is cooked through, about 5 to 7 minutes. With a slotted spatula, remove fish from the broth and place in a blender with the broccoli. Add cereal and blend until smooth.

Note: For older children, serve this dish in a scooped-out baked potato.

YIELD: 1–2 servings

Crispy Chicken Drummettes

4 chicken legs, or eight leggy portions of the chicken wing
1 cup milk-free bread crumbs
$1/2$ teaspoon garlic salt
$1/2$ teaspoon pepper
Milk-free margarine

Rinse chicken in cold water. Do not dry. Roll in milk-free bread crumbs. Place in a baking pan. Mix spices together and shake evenly over chicken. Dot each piece with a bit of milk-free margarine. Bake, uncovered, without turning at 375° for about 45 minutes.

YIELD: 2–4 servings

My Own Meat Loaf

Prepare your favorite meat loaf recipe, substituting calcium-fortified soy milk or other substitute for cow's milk. Many children prefer a lighter meat loaf composed of a blend of ground beef, mixed with ground veal or ground chicken or turkey. You may want to blend in an egg or some ketchup for moistness. Turn out the meat loaf preparation into individual loaf pans or into non-stick muffin tins. Bake about half or one-quarter the time a regular meat loaf takes to cook.

P and J on the Run

1 (8-inch) flour tortilla
2 tablespoons peanut butter
2 tablespoons jam or jelly
1 small banana, peeled

In the microwave, warm tortilla on a paper towel 10 to 20 seconds on high. Remove, and spread with peanut butter and jelly. Place the banana near the edge of the tortilla and fold up the bottom. Roll the banana into the tortilla. Voila!—a leakless peanut butter-and-jelly sandwich on the run.

YIELD: 1 serving

T and O Pasta

1 tablespoon vegetable oil
1/2 pound ground turkey
Salt and pepper to taste
1/2 cup cooked okra
1/2 cup tomato sauce
1 8-ounce portion of spaghetti or other pasta, cooked

In a sauté pan, brown the turkey in the oil. Drain. Add salt and pepper to taste. In a bowl, gently combine okra with tomato sauce. Pour into pan with browned turkey and cook on low heat for about 20 minutes. Serve over pasta.

YIELD: 2–4 servings

Microwave Wagon-Wheel Dinner

1 (16-ounce) can pork and beans
1 (8.5-ounce) can lima beans, rinsed and drained
1 (15-ounce) can red kidney beans, rinsed and drained
2 tablespoons minced onion
1/3 cup firmly packed brown sugar or 2 tablespoons blackstrap
    molasses
1 tablespoon prepared mustard
2 tablespoons barbecue sauce
6 milk-free turkey dogs

In a 2-quart glass casserole dish, combine pork and beans, lima beans, kidney beans, onion, brown sugar, mustard and barbecue sauce. Blend well. Cut each turkey dog in half and slit diagonally across the top, cutting in only about 1/4 inch. Arrange the turkey-dogs in a spoke design on top of the beans. Cover with plastic wrap, turning back a corner for steam release. Microwave on high for 12 to 15 minutes until the beans are bubbly and hot all

the way through. Rotate once during cooking. Let the dish stand
4 to 5 minutes to cool somewhat before serving.

YIELD: 4–6 servings

Tofu Scramble

Milk-free margarine
1 tablespoon chopped onion
Paprika
1 serving firm tofu, cubed
1 egg

In a small frying pan, melt margarine and sauté onion. Sprinkle
onion with paprika and cook until soft and golden. Toss in tofu
pieces. In a separate small bowl, beat egg until frothy and add to
pan. Scramble egg and tofu until cooked through and firmly set.
Serve on an English muffin with ham, stuff into a pita, or wrap in
a flour tortilla.

YIELD: 1 serving

Sloppy Josephines

$1/2$ pound ground turkey
$1/2$ pound lean ground beef
$1/4$ cup chopped green pepper
1 (10.75-ounce) can tomato soup
$1/4$ cup water
2 tablespoons minced onion
1 teaspoon prepared mustard
6 hamburger buns

In a sauté pan, brown ground turkey and beef until crumbly.
Drain off the fat. Add green pepper, tomato soup, water, onion
and mustard. Bring to a boil. Reduce heat and simmer for about
30 minutes. Serve on hamburger buns.

YIELD: 6 servings

Microwave Granola

$1/2$ cup milk-free margarine
$1/2$ cup honey
3 cups oats
$3/4$ cups sunflower seeds
1 cup chopped peanuts
$1/2$ cup wheat germ
$1/2$ cup brown sugar
$1/2$ cup raisins

In a small glass dish, microwave margarine on high for about 20 seconds or until melted. Remove and blend in the honey. In a large microwavable mixing bowl, combine oats, sunflower seeds, peanuts, wheat germ, and brown sugar. Add the melted margarine and honey and mix well with a wooden spoon. Microwave on high for about 4 minutes. Remove and stir. Microwave on high another 2 minutes. Add the raisins and stir. Microwave on high another 1 or 2 minutes or until the mixture is toasty. Remove and stir. Pour mixture out onto a cookie sheet and spread with the back of a wooden spoon. When it is cool, store in a covered container.

YIELD: About 6 cups

Fruits and Veggies

Hawaiian Casserole

2 egg whites
1 (16-ounce) can cut yams (drained)
1 cup crushed pineapple
Coconut

Beat egg whites until stiff. Set aside. In a large bowl, combine yams with pineapple. Add egg whites and blend gently. Pour into a greased 8-inch souffle dish. Bake at 350° for 20 minutes. Top with coconut and serve.

YIELD: 8 servings

Broccoli Noodle Casserole

8 ounces medium noodles
1 egg, slightly beaten
$3/4$ cup milk substitute (do not use juice)
1 envelope milk-free dry onion soup mix
4 tablespoons milk-free margarine, melted
1 (10-ounce) package frozen, chopped broccoli, thawed and drained

Cook noodles according to directions. Cook until tender but not soft. Remove and drain. In a large bowl, combine beaten egg and milk substitute with soup mix and melted margarine. Stir until well blended. Fold in broccoli and noodles. Pour into a $1^1/2$-quart casserole. Bake at 350° for 35 to 40 minutes. Remove from oven and let stand for about 10 minutes to set before serving.

YIELD: 4–6 servings

New Orleans Salad

1 small green pepper, chopped
1 small red pepper, chopped
1 small yellow pepper, chopped
$1/4$ pound fresh snow peas
1 large Boston lettuce
1 large Bibb lettuce

Chop peppers and set aside. Wash snow peas, remove strings if necessary, and set aside. Wash and dry lettuce. In salad bowl, blend vegetables. Top with Louisiana Dressing.

YIELD: 8 servings

LOUISIANA DRESSING

$^1/_2$ cup oil
$^1/_4$ cup red wine vinegar
1 tablespoon chopped red onion
2 teaspoons chopped chives
$^1/_4$ teaspoon salt
Dash of pepper

Blend these ingredients in a glass jar with a lid. Close lid and shake well.

Potato Stuffing

5 medium potatoes
$^1/_2$ teaspoon salt
$^1/_4$ cup milk-free margarine
$^1/_2$ cup chopped onion
$^1/_2$ cup chopped celery
2 cups milk-free bread crumbs
1 teaspoon salt
$^1/_2$ teaspoon pepper
1 egg, beaten

Peel potatoes and cut into quarters. Place potatoes and salt in a pot of boiling water and cook until tender, about 20 minutes. Drain well. Return potatoes to pot and mash until smooth. Over low heat, slowly stir potatoes until they are dry. In a separate saucepan, melt margarine and sauté onion and celery for about 5 minutes until tender. Add onion and celery mixture to potatoes. Add bread crumbs and seasonings. Beat with a wooden spoon until well mixed. Add beaten egg, and blend well. Bake at 350° in a greased, covered casserole dish 30 to 40 minutes, uncovering for the last 5 minutes for a browned top.

YIELD: 4–6 servings

Butternut Squash and Apple Bake

1 butternut squash (about 2 pounds)
$1/2$ cup brown sugar
$1/4$ cup melted milk-free margarine
1 tablespoon flour
1 teaspoon salt
$1/2$ teaspoon cinnamon
1 large apple, thinly sliced (your choice)

Cut squash in half, remove seeds and fiber. Cut off the skin, and cut squash into $1/2$-inch slices. In a small bowl, blend brown sugar, melted margarine, flour, salt, and cinnamon. Arrange squash slices in an ungreased 9-inch-square baking dish. Top with one half of the sugar/cinnamon mixture. Place a single layer of apple slices over the squash. Sprinkle the remaining sugar/cinnamon mixture over the top. Bake covered at 350° for 50 to 60 minutes or until the squash is tender. Uncover the last 5 to 8 minutes to brown.

YIELD: 6 servings

Cooked Greens

1 large bunch kale or collard greens, washed and chopped
1 large onion, chopped
1–2 cloves garlic, chopped
2 tablespoons oil
1 tablespoon flour
Salt and pepper to taste

Wash and chop greens, discarding all stems. Using a steamer, steam greens for about 20 minutes until tender. In a large saucepan, sauté onion and garlic in oil until tender. Add greens and the remaining ingredients. Toss well to blend.

YIELD: 4 servings

Nutty Banana Salad

2 (3-ounce) packages lemon gelatin (you may substitute
     sugar-free)
2 cups boiling water
1 1/4 cups cold water
3/4 cup sliced bananas
1/2 cup milk-free whipped-cream substitute
1/4 cup diced celery
1/4 cup chopped walnuts

In a mixing bowl, fully dissolve 1 package lemon gelatin in 1 cup
boiling water. Add 3/4 cup cold water and chill until thick. Add
bananas and spoon into a 6-cup mold and chill. In a mixing
bowl, fully dissolve 1 package lemon gelatin into 1 cup boiling
water. Add 3/4 cup cold water and chill until slightly thickened.
Blend in whipped-cream substitute, celery, and walnuts. Spoon
this mixture over clear gelatin mixture and chill until firm.

YIELD: 12 servings

Scalloped Potatoes

4 medium potatoes, peeled and sliced thinly
1 tablespoon flour
1 teaspoon salt
1/4 teaspoon pepper
1/4 teaspoon garlic powder
1 medium onion, sliced thinly
3/4 cup milk substitute (do not use juice)
2 tablespoons milk-free margarine
3/4 cup crushed dry cereal flakes or potato chips

Place a layer of potatoes in a greased casserole dish. In a small bowl, combine flour, salt, pepper, and garlic powder. Sprinkle about $1/2$ tablespoon of seasonings over potatoes. Add a layer of sliced onion. Add another layer of potatoes, seasonings, and onions until all ingredients are used. Pour milk substitute over the dish. Dot with margarine. Top with crushed dry cereal flakes or crushed potato chips. Bake at 375° for about 1 hour or longer until potatoes are tender.

YIELD: 4 servings

Mouthwatering Mashies

When making mashed potatoes, substitute any of the following for the milk:

Water in which the potatoes were cooked
Chicken broth
Beef broth
Milk substitutes such as soy milk or nondairy creamer
Consommé

To make potatoes extra fluffy, whip with an electric beater before serving.

Note: Here's a calcium-rich idea—blend mashed potatoes with cooked greens (collards, kale, spinach) for a swirly green vegetable–mashed potato dish. You might even stuff this mixture into prepared phyllo dough shells for a tasty finger-food snack or side dish. If you're really energetic, you could pour it from a pastry bag onto a cookie sheet and brown at 400° for just a few moments to make beautiful designs that are sure to be irresistible to kids.

Mexican Bean Salad

$1/2$ cup oil
$1/2$ cup prepared chili sauce
2 tablespoons cider vinegar
$1/2$ teaspoon salt
$1/4$ teaspoon pepper
2 red peppers, cored and cut into thin strips
$1 1/2$ pounds fresh green beans
1 (15.5-ounce) can garbanzo beans, washed and hulled
1 medium red onion, sliced
1 (5.75-ounce) can pitted black olives

In a mixing bowl, combine oil, chili sauce, vinegar, salt, pepper, and peppers. Set aside. Wash green beans and cut into 1-inch pieces. Steam or microwave until just soft—al dente. Drain beans and run under cold water to set. Place in a large bowl. Pour marinade over warm beans and add garbanzos, onions, and olives. Toss well. Cover with plastic wrap and refrigerate several hours or overnight.

YIELD: 6–8 servings

Traditional Tofu

2 tablespoons vegetable oil
$1/2$ pound soft tofu, crumbled
$1/2$ cup chopped broccoli
$1/2$ cup bok choy
1 tablespoon soy sauce

In a large frying pan or wok, heat oil until hot. Toss in tofu, broccoli, and bok choy. Brown well. Add soy sauce, reduce heat and simmer for about 2 minutes.

YIELD: 2–4 servings

Crispy Oniony Potatoes

4–6 medium-sized potatoes
1 tablespoon vegetable oil
1 package milk-free dry onion soup mix

Wash potatoes very well. Do not peel. Cut into 1-inch cubes. Toss
in a plastic bag with oil and onion soup mix. Bake in a 450° oven
for about 30 to 45 minutes, turning occasionally.

YIELD: 8 servings

Ramen Salad

$1/2$ head cabbage, shredded
1 small red onion, finely chopped
1 package ramen-type chicken-flavored noodles
$1/2$ cup slivered almonds
2 tablespoons sesame seeds
$1/2$ cup vinaigrette
1 teaspoon sugar
Salt and pepper to taste

Place shredded cabbage and chopped onion in a large bowl. On
a cookie sheet, break noodles into small pieces. Add almonds
and sesame seeds. Toast in a 300° oven for about 5 to 8 minutes
or until just lightly browned. In a small bowl, mix prepared vinaigrette with noodle seasoning packet, sugar, salt, and pepper to
taste. Add dressing to cabbage. Top with noodles, almonds, and
seeds. Toss well.

YIELD: 6–8 servings

Spinach Salad

12 ounces fresh spinach, washed, dried, and stems removed
1 pound cooked bacon
$^1/_2$ cup olive oil
$^1/_4$ cup tarragon vinegar
1 teaspoon dijon mustard
$^1/_2$ teaspoon sugar
Salt and pepper to taste
3 eggs, hard-boiled, shelled and sliced

In a large bowl, tear pieces of spinach and crumble the bacon. In
a small bowl, blend oil, vinegar, mustard, sugar, and salt and pepper to taste. Toss dressing through spinach and bacon. Garnish
with hard-boiled egg slices.

YIELD: 6 to 8 servings

Honey Baked Apple

4 medium-sized cooking apples
$^1/_3$ cup granola with raisins and nuts
1 teaspoon cinnamon
2 tablespoons honey
$^1/_2$ cup orange juice
2 tablespoons milk-free margarine

Wash the apples. Remove the cores and pare a 1-inch strip
around the top of each apple. Set the apples in a microwavable
baking dish. In a small bowl, combine granola with cinnamon
and honey. Spoon the mixture equally into the middle of each
apple. Pour the orange juice equally into each apple. Top each
one with milk-free margarine. Cover the apples with plastic wrap,
turning back a corner to vent. Microwave the apples on high for
4 minutes. Give the dish a half-turn. Microwave an additional 3
to 5 minutes, or until the apples are tender. Remove and let
stand 5 minutes more to set and cool.

YIELD: 4 servings

Fruit Roll

Use fresh apples, peaches, or pears. Wash and peel the fruit. Cook in a saucepan, adding sugar or honey, if you wish, for about 5 to 10 minutes, mashing the fruit as it cooks. Puree in a blender. Pour off excess water. On a cookie sheet, spread plastic wrap to cover. Spoon cooked fruit onto the wrap, staying away from the edges and spreading as thinly as possible. Spread another piece of plastic wrap over the mixture and press down with a wide spatula to even the mixture. Remove this top sheet of plastic and dry fruit in the oven on the lowest possible heat. A pilot light will do. Dry 6 to 8 hours or overnight. Remove, roll up the fruit and plastic wrap jelly-roll fashion. Slice into 3-inch pieces. Unroll and eat.

Red Hot and Cold Applesauce

1/4 cup cinnamon candies
1/2 cup water
1 (3-ounce) package red gelatin (raspberry or strawberry)
1 (16-ounce) jar natural applesauce

In a saucepan, over low heat, melt cinnamon candies in water until dissolved. Pour in the gelatin and continue to stir until gelatin is also melted. Remove from heat and add applesauce, combining well. Pour into individual glass dishes or a flat 8-inch glass baking pan. Refrigerate several hours until set.

YIELD: 6 servings.

Drinks

Calcium Hint: Looking for a way to boost your child's calcium intake? Why not crush one or two chewable calcium carbonate tablets and toss into juice or one of the fruit drinks below?

Morning Shake

1/2 cup calcium-fortified orange juice
1/2 cup milk substitute
1 large banana, sliced
3–6 ice cubes

Place all ingredients together in a blender. Blend at high speed until frothy.

YIELD: 1 serving

No, No, Nog

1/2 cup calcium-fortified orange juice
1/2 cup pineapple juice
1 egg
1 tablespoon honey
3–6 ice cubes

Mix all ingredients together in a blender. Blend at high speed until frothy. Do not serve if your child's pediatrician does not permit the eating of a raw egg.

YIELD: 1 serving

Hawaiian Sunrise

1 (8-ounce) can pineapple chunks in natural juice
3/4 cup calcium-fortified orange juice or papaya juice
4 maraschino cherries
3 ice cubes

Mix all ingredients together in a blender. Blend at high speed until frothy.

Yield: 1–2 servings

Carrot Cocktail

1 (8-ounce) can of sliced carrots
1/2 cup calcium-fortified orange juice
1/4 teaspoon ground cinnamon
2 tablespoons water
2 ice cubes

Do not drain carrots. Instead, blend all the ingredients including the liquid from the carrots together in a blender. Blend at high speed until smooth.

YIELD: 1–2 servings

Banana Berry Breakfast

1 whole ripe banana, sliced
1 cup frozen berries
1 cup apple juice
3 ice cubes

Mix all ingredients together in a blender. Blend at high speed until smooth.

YIELD: 1–2 servings

Tangy Watermelon Cooler

1/4 small watermelon
Juice of 1 lemon
Several ice cubes

Remove the watermelon rind and any seeds. Cut the melon into chunks and puree in a blender or food processor. Add lemon juice and pour over ice to serve.

YIELD: 1–2 servings

Snacks

Veggies and Curry Dip

Wash and drain an assortment of favorite raw vegetables. Prepare dip and serve as a meal or snack. Don't be surprised, lots of kids like the flavor of curry!

CURRY DIP

1 cup mayonnaise
1–2 teaspoons curry powder
2 tablespoons prepared chili sauce
2 teaspoons Worcestershire sauce
1/2 teaspoon garlic salt
Salt and pepper, if desired
1 teaspoon instant dried onion

Combine all ingredients and chill for 1 hour or more to let the flavors blend.

Tofu Dip

10.5 ounces soft tofu
1 packet milk-free dry ranch dressing mix or dry onion soup mix

In the blender, combine tofu, drained, with ranch dressing mix or dry onion soup mix. Serve with raw vegetables, chips, or triangles of pita bread.

Corn Muffins

1 (8.5-ounce) package milk-free corn muffin mix
1 (16.5-ounce) can creamed corn
1 egg

Blend all ingredients. Let batter rest about 5 minutes. Pour into a 12-cup muffin tin. Bake at 400° for 10 to 15 minutes. Serve warm.

YIELD: 12 muffins

Orange Custard

2 (10.5-ounce) packages of soft tofu, drained
$2/3$ cup calcium-enriched orange juice concentrate
1 tablespoon vegetable oil
1 teaspoon vanilla
2 tablespoons orange zest
3 tablespoons sugar or honey (optional)
Cinnamon

In a blender, combine tofu, orange juice concentrate, oil, vanilla, orange zest, and sugar, blending until thick and creamy. Pour mixture into ovenproof custard cups. Bake at 350° for about 30 minutes. Sprinkle with cinnamon. Serve hot.

Date and Nut Bread

1 (4-ounce) package pitted dates, cut into thirds
1 cup boiling water
$1^1/4$ cups flour
1 teaspoon baking soda
1 cup sugar
Dash salt
1 tablespoon milk-free margarine
1 egg, beaten
1 teaspoon vanilla extract
$3/4$ cup chopped nuts

Cover dates with boiling water and set aside. In a mixing bowl, sift flour, baking soda, sugar, and salt together. Mix in margarine and beaten egg. Beat until well blended. With a spoon, blend in date and water mixture. Stir until the batter is moistened. Stir in vanilla and nuts. Turn into a well-greased loaf pan. Bake at 350° for about 45 minutes.

YIELD: 1 loaf

Bran Muffins

1^1/$_2$ cups 100-percent wheat bran cereal
^{1}/$_2$ cup boiling water
^{1}/$_2$ cup sugar
^{1}/$_4$ cup vegetable oil
1 egg
1 cup soy milk or other milk substitute
1^1/$_4$ cups flour
1^1/$_4$ teaspoons baking soda
^{1}/$_4$ teaspoon salt

Add ^{1}/$_2$ cup bran cereal to boiling water and soak. In another bowl, cream sugar and vegetable oil. Add egg and blend until mixture is light yellow. Add soy milk and beat well. Fold in remaining dry bran cereal and mix until moist. In another bowl, sift together flour, baking soda, and salt. Add the dry ingredients and the bran/water mixture to the batter. Stir until combined. Do not overmix. Pour into greased muffin cups until ^{2}/$_3$ full. Bake at 350° for 20 to 25 minutes or until golden brown.

YIELD: 12 muffins

Eggless Apple Muffins

1 cup unbleached flour
1 cup whole wheat flour
^{1}/$_2$ cup sugar
2 tablespoons wheat germ
1 tablespoon baking powder
^{1}/$_4$ teaspoon nutmeg
1 cup peeled, grated, apple
^{1}/$_2$ cup raisins
1 cup apple juice
^{1}/$_3$ cup oil
Egg substitute: ^{1}/$_2$ teaspoon baking powder and 2 tablespoons juice

2 tablespoons sugar
$1/4$ teaspoon cinnamon

Line a muffin pan with paper baking cups or generously grease 12 muffin cups. In a large bowl, combine flours with sugar, wheat germ, baking powder, and nutmeg. Add apple and raisins. Stir in apple juice, oil, and egg substitute until moistened. Spoon batter into prepared muffin cups, filling three-quarters full. In a small bowl, blend sugar and cinnamon. Sprinkle over batter. Bake at 400° for 20 to 25 minutes or until golden brown. Let set at least 1 hour before eating.

YIELD: 12 muffins

Oatmeal Banana Bread

$1/2$ cup vegetable shortening
$1/2$ cup sugar
2 eggs
1 cup unbleached flour
1 teaspoon baking soda
$1/4$ teaspoon salt
$1/2$ teaspoon cinnamon
$1 1/2$ cups mashed bananas
$1/4$ cup milk substitute or applesauce
1 cup quick or regular oatmeal
1 cup raisins

In a large bowl, cream shortening and sugar. Add eggs and beat until very creamy. In a separate bowl, blend flour, baking soda, salt, and cinnamon. Gradually add to creamed mixture, beating thoroughly. Alternately, add bananas and milk substitute to batter. Stir in oatmeal and raisins. Pour into a greased loaf pan. Bake at 350° for about 1 hour.

YIELD: 1 loaf

Rice Cake-a-Mania

Top mini rice cakes with one of these great food ideas for a healthy snack.

> Salmon spread
> Tuna spread
> Peanut butter and jelly
> Peanut butter and banana
> Cold cuts
> Egg salad
> Shrimp salad
> Sautéed tofu slices
> Apple butter
> Almond butter

The Zukin Dip

This dish is a favorite of my family's and all of our friends who share the kitchen table with us. It is a treat I always make for my daughter when she comes home from college and has become a Zukin tradition. You may have eaten something like this which has been made with sour cream and shredded cheese. But I guarantee you won't miss the dairy products in this version.

1 can vegetarian refried beans
3 ripe avocados, peeled and pitted
2–3 tablespoons orange juice
2 large tomatoes, chopped
1 can pitted black olives, chopped
1 can chopped mild chiles
$1/2$ cup chopped green onion
Tortilla chips

In a 9-by-13-inch glass pan, spread refried beans along the bottom as the first layer of the dip. In a small bowl, mash avocados.

Add orange juice to avocados to make a spreadable consistency. Adjust the amount of juice accordingly. Spread avocado mixture over the refried beans. Layer with chopped tomatoes, olives, and chilis. Top with chopped green onion. Refrigerate for about 30 minutes to allow the flavors to set. Serve with tortilla chips.

Fruit Kebabs

Using small wooden skewers, alternate pieces of freshly cut fruit in season. For a Winter/Fall Kebab, use chunks of banana, apple, orange. For a Spring/Summer Kebab, use chunks of melon, seedless grapes, strawberries.

Crunchy Blend of Goodness

In a large bowl with a tight cover, blend a variety of bite-sized milk-free crunchy and sweet foods such as pretzels, popcorn, oyster crackers, almonds, peanuts, enriched dry cereal (round ones and square ones), dried fruit, cut-up figs or dates, and raisins. Scoop out this snack as desired or fill small plastic bags for quick and easy access. Makes a nice accompaniment to a brown-bag lunch.

Mild Guacamole with Jicama

2 soft avocados, peeled and pitted
1/4 cup calcium-fortified orange juice
1 green onion, finely chopped (optional)
1 tomato, chopped
1 large jicama, peeled and julienned

In a small bowl, mash avocados well. Add orange juice and green onion. Blend well. Top with chopped tomato. Refrigerate at least 30 minutes to let flavors set. Serve with jicama strips or corn chips.

YIELD: 8 servings

Frozen Juice Pops

Freeze calcium-fortified juice in an ice-cube tray. Toss into other juices or soft drinks to enrich them. Or make frozen pops by pressing in wooden pops sticks when mixture is almost frozen, but still soft enough to hold the sticks.

Hummus with Pita

1 (15-ounce) can garbanzo beans, rinsed and drained
2 tablespoons chopped chives
2 cloves garlic, minced
1 tablespoon olive oil
3 tablespoons lemon juice
$1/2$ teaspoon salt
$1/4$ teaspoon white pepper

Place all ingredients in a food processor or blender. Puree, adding water if needed. Chill at least 1 hour before serving. Serve with triangles of pita bread. Hummus also makes a terrific sandwich spread instead of mayonnaise or as the sandwich filling itself.

Little Renee's Favorite Sunshine

2 tablespoons peanut butter
1 Granny Smith apple, sliced and cored

Swirl peanut butter in a beautiful circle in the center of a small plate. Surround the peanut butter with apple slices like the rays of the sun.

YIELD: 1 serving

Black Bean Salsa

1 (15-ounce) can black beans, rinsed and drained
$1/2$ cup frozen corn, defrosted
$1/2$ cup prepared mild salsa
1 tablespoon chopped fresh parsley
1 tablespoon chopped fresh cilantro
8 romaine lettuce leaves, rinsed and dried

In a bowl, blend beans, corn, salsa, parsley, and cilantro. Refrigerate for about 30 minutes to let flavors blend. Prepare lettuce leaves and arrange on a serving plate. Scoop out some salsa on each lettuce leaf to serve.

YIELD: 8 servings

Treats

Milk-Free Vanilla Ice Cream

1 (8-ounce) container Rich's Richwhip Frozen Non-Dairy
      Whipping Cream
$1/2$ cup sugar
1 teaspoon vanilla
1 egg (separated)

Chill beaters and bowl in the freezer for 10 minutes before starting. Whip thawed topping for 2 minutes. Add sugar, vanilla, and egg yolk, and freeze for 30 minutes. In a small bowl, beat egg white until stiff. Remove ice cream from freezer, fold in egg white, and beat for 1 minute. Pour into plastic container, cover, and freeze. Ice cream will be ready in 24 hours. Makes 1 quart.

Note: My sources assure me that freezing raw egg kills any unwanted bacteria. However, if you are concerned, you should check with your child's pediatrician before serving this recipe.

YIELD: 8 servings

VARIATIONS

Chocolate Ice Cream   Add $1/4$ cup cocoa powder to ice cream before freezing for the first 30 minutes.

Nutty Buddy Ice Cream   Add chopped nuts and milk-free semi-sweet chocolate morsels to ice cream before freezing for the final time.

Cookie Ice Cream   Add broken cookie pieces to the ice cream before freezing for the final time.

Tutti-Frutti Ice Cream   Add 1 cup frozen fruit (drained) to ice cream before freezing for the first 30 minutes. Fresh fruit can also be added, but may require additional sugar.

Milk-Free Ice Cream Toppers

Hershey's Syrup

Strawberry sauce

Pineapple sauce

Raspberry sauce

Marshmallow sauce

Milk-free whipped cream

Sliced bananas

Pieces of dried apple, pineapple, apricot

Granola

Trail mix

Sugar sprinkles

Colored sugar

Fresh fruit bits

Fruit or Vegetable Sorbet

Sorbet may be made in just about any flavor—watermelon, cantaloupe, strawberry, raspberry, carrot, pumpkin. Use your imagination.

3 cups fruit or vegetable puree
1 cup sorbet syrup
or
2 cups fruit juice
2 cups syrup

Add puree or juice to chilled syrup (syrup recipe follows). Pour into a 9-inch metal cake pan and freeze for 30 minutes. Remove and thaw for 10 minutes. Pour into a chilled bowl. Beat mixture for 3 minutes. Scoop into paper-lined muffin cups and freeze.

YIELD: 1 quart—8 servings.

SORBET SYRUP

$2/3$ cup water
$2/3$ cup sugar

Combine water and sugar in a small saucepan. Stir over medium heat until sugar is dissolved. Do not let mixture boil. Pour syrup into a mixing bowl and chill thoroughly.

YIELD: 1 cup.

Milk-Free Parfait

1 serving of milk-free ice cream
3 crushed cookies of your choice
2 tablespoons milk-free whipped cream
1 tablespoon chopped nuts
2 maraschino cherries

Put $1/2$ of the ice cream in a parfait glass. Top with $1/2$ of the crushed cookies, followed by the remaining ice cream and the remaining cookies. Top with whipped cream, nuts, and the cherries.

YIELD: 1 serving.

continues

Other milk-free parfait toppers:

Chopped dates
Raisins
Chopped figs
Dried apricots
Banana slices
Kiwi slices
Melon balls
Sunflower seeds
Mandarin orange slices

Mini Pumpkin Pies

2 (9-inch) prepared pie shells (unbaked)
Nonstick cooking spray
2 eggs, beaten slightly
1 (16-ounce) can pumpkin
$3/4$ cup sugar
$1/2$ teaspoon salt
2 teaspoons cinnamon
1 teaspoon nutmeg
8 ounces milk substitute (do not use juice)
Optional: milk-free whipped cream

On a very lightly floured board, roll out pie crusts just slightly to $1/8$-inch thickness. With a $2^1/2$-inch glass or cookie cutter, cut out rounds of crust. Spray a $1^1/2$-inch tart shell pan with nonstick cooking spray. Place a crust in each tart shell cup and crimp as you would a pie crust. Set aside. To prepare filling, combine eggs with remaining ingredients until well blended. Fill each mini pie to the top. Bake at 425° for 10 minutes. Turn down the heat to 350° and continue baking for about 15 to 20 minutes or until an inserted toothpick comes out clean. Remove and let cool thoroughly. Top with a dollop of milk-free whipped cream if desired.

YIELD: 36 mini pies

Peanut Butter Puff Bars

$1/4$ cup milk-free margarine
$1/4$ cup peanut butter
10 ounces marshmallows
6 cups puffed rice or wheat cereal

Grease a 15-by-10-inch jelly roll pan. Over double boiler, melt margarine, combined with peanut butter and marshmallows. Let cool slightly. Remove from heat. Add puffed cereal and press into pan. Chill and slice into bars.

YIELD: 36 bars

Variation: Drizzle with melted milk-free chocolate

Hot Peach Angel Cake

3 tablespoons sugar
2 teaspoons cornstarch
$1/2$ cup water
Pinch ground nutmeg
2 large peaches, pared and sliced
$1/4$ teaspoon almond extract
1 prepared angel food cake

In a small saucepan, combine sugar, cornstarch, water, and nutmeg, stirring until smooth. Add peaches and cook over medium heat, stirring constantly until mixture boils. Boil for about 1 minute. Remove from heat. Stir in almond extract. Serve warm over angel food cake.

YIELD: $1\,1/2$ cups

Raspberry Chocolate Pudding

1 (8-ounce) package chocolate soy drink
$^1/_2$ pound silken tofu, crumbled
$^3/_4$ cup raspberries
1 medium banana
1 tablespoon honey
2 teaspoons cocoa powder
$^1/_4$ teaspoon cinnamon

Place soy drink, tofu, $^1/_2$ cup raspberries, banana, honey, cocoa powder, and cinnamon in a blender and blend until smooth. Pour into 4 stemmed glasses and refrigerate for one hour or more, until mixture is set. Top with remaining raspberries and serve immediately.

Yield: 4 servings

Old-Fashioned Apple Cake

$^1/_2$ stick milk-free margarine, melted
6 apples (your choice) peeled, cored, and sliced
1 tablespoon lemon juice
1 tablespoon cinnamon
$^2/_3$ cup sugar
2 eggs, beaten
1 cup unbleached flour
2 teaspoons baking powder
1 teaspoon vanilla extract
1 teaspoon almond extract
$^1/_2$ cup chopped walnuts (optional)

Pour margarine in a 9-inch-square baking pan and set aside. In a large bowl, mix together apples, lemon juice, cinnamon, and $^1/_3$ cup sugar. Pour into pan. In a mixing bowl, blend eggs, $^1/_3$ cup sugar, flour, baking powder, and vanilla and almond extracts.

Spread this mixture over the apples. Top with chopped nuts, if desired. Blend this mixture with a knife. Bake at 350° for about 45 minutes.

YIELD: 8–12 servings

Cinnamon Nut Pastry Roll

1 (9-inch) prepared pie crust
2 tablespoons applesauce
2 tablespoons packed brown sugar
3 tablespoons chopped nuts
$1/2$ teaspoon ground cinnamon
1 tablespoon milk-free margarine

Roll out pastry to 14-by-8-inch rectangle. Place on an ungreased cookie sheet. Spread with applesauce. In a small bowl, mix brown sugar, nuts, and cinnamon. Sprinkle this mixture over the applesauce. Starting at one end, roll the pastry tightly. Pinch in the ends to seal. Bake at 425° for 9 to 11 minutes. Slice and serve.

YIELD: 8 servings

Chocolate Fondue

$2/3$ cup light corn syrup
$1/2$ cup milk substitute
8 squares (ounces) baking chocolate
$1/2$ cup each: strawberries, sliced kiwi, pineapple chunks, apple chunks, banana chunks

In a small saucepan, cook and blend corn syrup with milk substitute until boiling. Remove from heat. Add chocolate squares and blend until melted smooth. Transfer to a heated fondue pot, or serve in individual bowls. Dip the fruit in the chocolate and enjoy.

Frozen Fruit Slush

$1/2$ (6-ounce) can frozen lemonade concentrate
$1/2$ cup orange juice
$1/2$ cup lemon-lime soda
1 cup crushed pineapple with juice
1 cup fresh raspberries
1 cup fresh strawberries, sliced
2 bananas, thinly sliced

In a blender, whip all ingredients until frothy. Pour into a 9-inch-square pan. Freeze for 2 to 3 hours or until firm, but still slushy. Serve in parfait glasses.

YIELD: 8 servings

Orange Bars

2 egg yolks
1 cup solid shortening (milk-free margarine may be used)
$3/4$ cup sugar
1 teaspoon vanilla
$1/2$ teaspoon salt
$2 1/4$ cups flour
Orange marmalade

In a mixing bowl, combine egg yolks, shortening, sugar, vanilla, and salt. Add flour slowly until a dough is formed. Divide the dough into three balls and refrigerate for several hours or overnight. Lightly grease a 9-by-13-inch baking pan. Grate the dough into the pan from 2 of the dough balls. Cover with orange marmalade. Grate the dough from the third ball on top. Bake at 350° for 15 minutes or until golden brown. Cut into squares while hot.

YIELD: 24–48 squares

Baby Lemon Tarts

24 tart crusts
$1/3$ cup milk-free margarine
1 cup sugar
1 teaspoon lemon rind
$1/3$ cup lemon juice
$1/4$ teaspoon salt
4 egg yolks

Melt margarine on top of a double boiler. Add sugar, lemon rind, lemon juice, salt, and yolks, which have been beaten slightly in a bowl. Cook over boiling water about 10 minutes, stirring constantly. Cool until thickened. Pour into cooled tart shells.

YIELD: 24 tarts

TART CRUSTS

$1^1/2$ cups flour
$1/2$ teaspoon salt
$1/2$ cup solid shortening or milk-free margarine
3–4 tablespoons cold water

In a mixing bowl, blend flour with salt. Cut in shortening until the mixture is the size of small peas. Sprinkle cold water over the mixture, turning lightly with a fork until dough is moist enough to hold together. Form into a ball. Roll out on a floured board to $1/8$-inch thickness. Cut into rounds with a $3^1/2$-inch cookie cutter. Press rounds into a small 24-count muffin tin and prick the rounds with a fork. Bake at 450° 10 to 12 minutes or until lightly browned. Remove to cool and fill.

No-Bake Toffee Squares

3 eggs, separated
1 cup crushed milk-free vanilla wafers
1 cup chopped pecans
1/2 cup milk-free margarine, softened
1 cup confectioners' sugar
1 1/2 squares baking chocolate, melted
1/2 teaspoon vanilla

In a small bowl, beat the egg whites until stiff. Set aside. In a mixing bowl, blend the vanilla wafers and pecans together. Using half the wafer/nut mixture, cover the bottom of a greased 9-inch-square baking pan. In a small bowl, cream the margarine and sugar. Add egg yolks and beat until creamy. Add the melted chocolate and vanilla and blend well. Slowly fold in the stiffly beaten egg whites, blending well. Pour this mixture over the wafer/nut crust and sprinkle remaining wafer/nut mixture on top. Refrigerate overnight. Cut into squares.

YIELD: 12–16 squares.

Healthy Strawberry Pie

1/2–3/4 cup sugar
2 tablespoons cornstarch
2 tablespoons light corn syrup
1 cup water
2 tablespoons strawberry gelatin powder
1 quart fresh, whole strawberries, washed and trimmed
1 prepared 9-inch pie shell

In a small pot, mix the sugar, cornstarch, syrup, and water together. Bring mixture to a boil and cook until thick and clear. Add the gelatin and stir until dissolved. Set aside to cool. In the pie shell, arrange the whole berries to cover the bottom. (Berries may be sliced if you wish.) Pour the gelatin mixture over the berries and chill until set.

Yield: 8 servings

Nutty Chocolate Marshmallows

1 (6-ounce) package milk-free semisweet chocolate morsels
2 tablespoons milk-free margarine
1 egg, slightly beaten
1 cup confectioners' sugar
2 cups miniature marshmallows
1 cup ground nuts (your choice)

Melt chocolate morsels and margarine over low heat. Remove and blend in egg. Add sugar and marshmallows, blending well. Shape into 1-inch balls. Roll in nuts and chill.

YIELD: 3 dozen clusters

Banana Peanut Cookies

1 1/4 cup flour
1 1/2 teaspoons baking powder
1/2 teaspoon salt
1/3 cup brown sugar
1/3 cup sugar
1/2 cup vegetable oil
1/2 cup peanut butter
1 banana, mashed
1/2 cup peanuts

Mix all ingredients with an electric mixer. Drop by teaspoonfuls onto a cookie sheet. Bake 10 to 12 minutes at 375°.

YIELD: 2 dozen cookies

Chocolate Peanut Brittle

1 cup sugar
1/2 cup shelled peanuts, chopped
2 pinches salt
1/2 cup milk-free semisweet chocolate morsels
1 tablespoon milk-free margarine

Melt sugar over low heat until golden brown. Remove from heat and add nuts and salt. Blend well. Pour onto a greased cookie sheet, thinly covering. While this mixture cools, melt chocolate morsels and margarine. Combine and drizzle over peanut brittle. Let cool thoroughly. Break into bite-size pieces.

YIELD: serves 2–4

Sprinkly Oatmeal-Lemon Bars

4 sticks milk-free margarine, softened
1 cup sugar
2 cups unbleached flour
3 cups uncooked oatmeal (quick or regular)
1 tablespoon lemon zest
1 teaspoon vanilla
Confectioners' sugar
Sugar sprinkles (multicolored or chocolate)

In a large bowl, cream margarine and sugar. Add flour, oatmeal, lemon zest, and vanilla. Blend well with a wooden spoon. Cover and chill about 30 minutes. Shape dough into 1-inch balls and place on an ungreased cookie sheet. Flatten with the bottom of a glass that has been dipped in the confectioners' sugar. Bake at 350° for 12 to 15 minutes or until edges are light brown. Cool 1 minute on the cookie sheet before removing to a wire rack. Top with colorful sugar sprinkles.

YIELD: 4 dozen cookies

Rocky Road Bars

$1/4$ cup flour
$1/4$ teaspoon baking powder
$1/8$ teaspoon salt
$1/3$ cup dark brown sugar, packed
1 egg
1 tablespoon milk-free margarine, softened
$1/2$ teaspoon vanilla
1 cup coarsely chopped walnuts
1 cup large marshmallows, cut into quarters
6 ounces milk-free semisweet chocolate morsels

In a large mixing bowl, blend flour with baking powder and salt. Add sugar, egg, margarine, and vanilla. Beat until creamy smooth. Stir in $1/2$ cup walnuts. Turn into a lightly greased 9-inch-square baking pan. Bake at 350° for 15 minutes until the top is lightly browned and springs back when touched gently with your finger. Remove from the oven. Immediately arrange the marshmallows on top and sprinkle on the remaining walnuts and chocolate morsels. Return the pan to the oven for about 2 minutes, or just until the chocolate is softened. Remove from the oven and with a knife or spatula, swirl the chocolate over the marshmallows and walnuts. Cool until the chocolate is set. Cut into squares.

YIELD: 16 squares.

Microwave S'Mores

1 whole milk-free graham cracker
1 large marshmallow
$1/2$ bar milk-free dark chocolate

Break the graham cracker into 2 pieces. Place the chocolate bar on top of 1 piece, top with a marshmallow and microwave on high for about 10 seconds. Top with the second graham cracker and squash the sandwich together while the chocolate and marshmallow are hot.

YIELD: 1 serving

My Pie

1 (21-ounce) can fruit pie filling
1/2 cup firmly packed brown sugar
1/3 cup flour
1/3 cup quick rolled oats   .
3 tablespoons milk-free margarine, melted

Spoon pie filling evenly into 5 glass custard cups. In a small bowl, combine brown sugar, flour, and oats until well blended. Add melted milk-free margarine and toss with a fork until crumbly. Sprinkle this topping over each fruit-filled custard cup. Place the custard cups in the microwave in a circle. Microwave on high for about 3 1/2 minutes. Give the cups a quarter turn. Microwave on high for 2 to 3 minutes until the tops are toasty and the fruit filling is bubbly. Carefully remove and let cool for several minutes before serving. Make sure the centers are not too hot.

YIELD: 5 servings

Sticky Buns

1 loaf milk-free frozen bread dough
1/4 cup milk-free margarine
1/3 cup brown sugar
1/3 cup blackstrap molasses
1/2 cup chopped nuts

Thaw bread dough. In a small pot, melt margarine. Add brown sugar and molasses and cook on very low heat until dissolved and blended. Pour this mixture into a greased 8-inch-square baking pan. Sprinkle chopped nuts over the mixture. Shape bread dough into 9 or 12 balls and place in the pan. Let bread rise at room temperature to the top of the pan. Bake at 350° for 30 minutes. Cool 3 minutes, then invert on plate.

YIELD: 9–12 servings

Oatmeal Peanut Butter Chewies

$1/2$ cup milk-free margarine
$1 1/2$ cups brown sugar
2 eggs
$1/2$ cup chunky peanut butter
$1 1/2$ cups quick rolled oats
1 cup flour

In a bowl, cream margarine and brown sugar until light and fluffy. Beat in eggs. Add peanut butter and blend well. Add oats and flour, mixing well. Turn out into a 9-by-13-inch baking pan and bake at 325° for 35 minutes. Cool and cut into squares.

YIELD: about 36 squares

Brown-Bagging

Here are some hints for making brown-bagging safe and enjoyable.

Food is best kept refrigerated, which may be accomplished in a variety of ways. You might want to purchase small, reusable ice packs, which can be found in supermarkets or stores that sell camping supplies. You can also freeze individual containers of fruit juice or juice boxes to act as a refrigerant for the packed meal. They should thaw in plenty of time to drink while keeping the meal very cold. Remember to enclose the freezing element in a plastic bag if your child will be using an actual brown bag to carry her lunch. If your child can eat yogurt, it may be frozen and packed into the sack as well, although it must be blended a little bit before eating if any separation has taken place.

If your child will be carrying a Thermos for hot foods, it must be periodically checked to be sure that it is maintaining a temperature of at least 140° Fahrenheit until lunchtime to prevent bacterial growth. Some suggest filling the Thermos with very hot water and letting it stand for a few minutes, then dumping the water out and refilling the Thermos with the soup or other food to be carried for lunch. This method preheats the Thermos to the correct temperature.

Always use new plastic bags for packing food. Reusing bread or grocery store produce bags may transfer bacteria to your child's lunch. Also, avoid using bags with printed lettering because the ink may contain lead and flake off onto the food. If your child is using a lunchbox, choose one that is easy to clean, perhaps one that is dishwasher safe. Allow it to dry completely before each use. If your child insists on a metal lunchbox, you would probably do best to wrap all her foods in individual plastic bags, which can be well sealed.

Tortilla Wrap-Ups

Instead of a sandwich, use a soft flour tortilla to wrap meats and vegetables. Spread the ingredients on the tortilla and roll it up. Using more than one ingredient in the tortilla makes the finished product look colorful and interesting. Fasten with a toothpick or tie with long chives. Try these combinations:

Turkey, ham, lettuce, mayo

Hummus, shredded lettuce

Salmon spread, sliced olives

Tuna salad, sweet pickle relish

Liver pate, hard-boiled egg

Egg salad, cooked cold asparagus

Chicken salad, chopped cooked broccoli

Ratatouille

Chopped shrimp, salsa

Sliced cooked chicken, cooked greens (collards, spinach)

Stir-fried tofu strips

Meat Loaf Dogs

The perfect way to use leftover meat loaf. Cut a slice of meat loaf vertically, in the shape of a hot dog. Place in a hot-dog bun and top with whatever fixins' your child likes—ketchup, mustard, relish, onion. For some reason, the novelty makes this cold sandwich extremely appetizing.

Pasta Heaven

Prepare your child's favorite compact pasta noodles such as shells, rings, rotini. Be sure to rinse with cold water after cooking. Add cold vegetables such as broccoli florets, chopped green pepper, chopped tomatoes, or bits of chicken, turkey, fish, or sliced hard-boiled egg. Blend with a touch of vinaigrette. Make sure it is carried in a leak-proof container.

Your Very Own Lunch-ibles

Wrap six or eight crackers in plastic wrap. Cut six or eight pieces of ham or turkey bologna to fit the crackers exactly, and wrap these in plastic wrap. Do the same with six or eight slices of soy cheese (if tolerated). Toss these into a plastic bag together with a little bag of popcorn or pretzels. Voila! Almost the same kind of snazzy lunch pack as the ones sold in the supermarket refrigerated sections.

Souper Thermos

Fill your child's Thermos with her favorite hearty soup. You might want to toss in a few slices of turkey dogs or chunks of chicken for an added protein source. If your child likes chili, it stays warm in a Thermos as well.

Whatever on Wheat Bread

A healthy sandwich starts with healthy bread. For children who can tolerate wheat, whole-wheat bread provides some vitamins, minerals, fiber, and protein. Whatever you put on whole-wheat bread is made that much more nutritious. For children who don't care for the flavor, try using sandwich ingredients that have a strong flavor of their own, for example mustard as a spread instead of mayonnaise or sugar-cured ham instead of boiled ham.

Begg-al

Scramble an egg in the morning for your child to take for lunch that afternoon. Top with a tomato, and stuff it inside a bagel. Secure tightly in plastic wrap. Make sure your child's brown bag contains a frozen ice pack to preserve freshness.

Veggy 'n' Dip Lunch

Prepare a variety of raw vegetables for your child to dip in a tofu-based dip. The tofu provides calcium and protein, while the vegetables provide the vitamins and minerals. You will need a well-sealed container for the dip. A bagel or hunk of French bread complements the meal nicely.

Salad on a Stick

On 2 small wooden skewers, alternate cherry tomatoes, chunks of zucchini, cucumber, broccoli, tofu, cooked chicken, cooked turkey, or cubed ham. Toss in a plastic bag with a little vinaigrette. The skewered salad will be marinated perfectly by lunchtime.

Beef 'n' Pita

¹/2 pita bread round
1 serving cold roast beef
1 teaspoon ketchup
1 teaspoon mayonnaise
Shredded lettuce

Chop the roast beef. In a small bowl blend the ketchup and mayonnaise. Add roast beef and blend. Stuff the pita and top with shredded lettuce. Wrap tightly in plastic wrap.

Vegetarian Taco Roll-Up

On a soft flour tortilla, spread a thick layer of refried beans. Top with chopped olives, chopped tomatoes, chopped green chiles. Top with taco sauce and shredded lettuce. Fold in the sides and roll up. Can be served hot or cold.

Birthday Party Ideas

For many children, a birthday party is the essence of their social life. They need not be left out of the fun just because they cannot have dairy foods. It is always a good idea to keep some milk-free frosted cupcakes in the freezer for your child to take along to a party he or she might attend. However, when it is your turn to host a dairy-free birthday party for your child, you will have these party ideas to use as a starting point. They are meant to spur your imagination. I am sure that many of you are much more creative than I am in this department, but here are a few basics. By the way, each party idea comes with a wonderful cake recipe. If you wish to add milk-free ice cream you can make your own (see recipes in the Treats section) or purchase one of several varieties on the market, such as Mocha Mix, Rice Dream, or Tofutti.

The Western Roundup

Menu:

Franks and beans

Wagon wheel noodles (wheel-shaped pasta)

Applesauce in the can (cover individual containers of applesauce in aluminum foil)

Pineapple Upside-Down Cake (below)

Pineapple Upside-Down Cake—A Frontier Favorite

3 tablespoons milk-free margarine
3/4 cup brown sugar
1 (8.5-ounce) can sliced pineapple in light syrup (reserve syrup)
1/3 cup milk-free margarine, softened
1/2 cup sugar
1 egg
1 1/2 teaspoons vanilla
1 cup flour
1 1/2 teaspoons baking powder
1/4 teaspoon salt

In a small pan, melt 3 tablespoons milk-free margarine. Add brown sugar and 1 tablespoon pineapple juice. Set aside. In a large bowl, cream together 1/3 cup milk-free margarine and sugar. Add egg and vanilla, and beat until fluffy. In another bowl, sift together flour, baking powder, and salt. Add to creamed mixture alternating with remaining pineapple syrup. Using an 8-inch-square baking pan, pour in brown sugar and margarine mixture. Arrange pineapple slices in the pan and cover with batter. Bake at 350° for about 40 minutes. Cool 5 minutes and invert onto a serving plate.

YIELD: 9 servings

A Pastel Party

Menu:

Corn Chowder (page 278)

Open-faced salmon or ham spread on white bread triangles

Fruit cocktail

Pastel Cake with Sprinkles (below)

Pastel Cake with Sprinkles

1 package milk-free white cake mix
2 cups boiling water
1 large package cherry gelatin
Pastel sugar sprinkles

Prepare cake according to directions on the package in a 9-by-13-inch baking pan. At $3/2$-inch intervals, poke holes in the cake with a large fork. Prepare gelatin in the following manner: Pour boiling water into the mix and stir until gelatin is dissolved. Carefully pour the red gelatin over the cake. Refrigerate for at least 3 hours or overnight. To remove from pan, dip the cake pan in warm water about 10 seconds and turn out onto a serving plate. Top with pastel sugar sprinkles. Keep refrigerated until ready to serve.

YIELD: 12 servings

All-American Party

Menu:

Hamburger on a bun

Assorted condiments including ketchup, mustard, relish, pickles,
    sliced tomatoes, shredded lettuce

French fries

Carrot sticks

Celery sticks

Chocolate Cake with Chocolate Frosting (below)

Chocolate Cake with Chocolate Frosting

$2/3$ cup milk-free margarine

$1\,2/3$ cups sugar

3 eggs

$1/2$ teaspoon vanilla

2 cups flour

$2/3$ cup cocoa powder

$1\,1/4$ teaspoons baking soda

1 teaspoon salt

$1/4$ teaspoon baking powder

$1\,1/3$ cups water

In a large mixing bowl, combine margarine, sugar, eggs, and vanilla. Beat on high for 3 minutes. In a separate bowl, combine flour, cocoa powder, baking soda, salt, and baking powder. Add alternately with water to creamed mixture. Beat well. Pour into 2 greased 9-inch round baking pans. Bake at 350° for 30 to 35 minutes. Let cakes cool in pans for 10 minutes. Invert onto wire racks to cool completely before frosting.

YIELD: 12–16 servings

CHOCOLATE FROSTING

3 cups confectioners' sugar

$3/4$ cup cocoa powder

Pinch salt

2 teaspoons vanilla

$1/3$ cup milk-free margarine, softened

5 tablespoons milk substitute (do not use juice)

In a mixing bowl, combine sugar, cocoa powder, salt, vanilla, and margarine, beating well. Slowly add milk substitute until frosting is of spreading consistency. Add additional milk substitute or water if necessary.

Make-Your-Own Party

Menu:

My Very Own Meatloaf (page 289)

Twice-stuffed potato with assorted toppings (bake large potatoes, cut in half, scoop out and mash the potatoes, then stuff back into potato skins)

Assorted toppings including crumbled bacon, chopped ham, chopped green pepper, chopped tomato, salsa, chili

Fruit Kebabs (page 309)

Decorate-Your-Own Cupcakes (below)

Decorate-Your-Own Cupcakes

$1/2$ cup milk-free margarine, softened
$1 1/2$ cups sifted flour
$3/4$ cup sugar
$2 1/2$ teaspoons baking powder
$1/2$ teaspoon salt
1 egg
$3/4$ cup water
$1 1/2$ teaspoons vanilla

In a large bowl, blend margarine, flour, sugar, baking powder, and salt. Add egg and $1/2$ the water, and mix until just moist. Beat at medium speed until well blended. Add the rest of the water and vanilla. Beat again. Bake in 8 paper-lined muffin cups at 375° for about 15 minutes. Frost when cool.

YIELD: 8 servings

Topping Assortment:

Sugar sprinkles

Jelly beans

Milk-free semisweet chocolate morsels

Licorice bits

Dried fruit bits

Soft fruit candies

Red Hots

Perfect Picnic Birthday

Menu:

Pack in individual baskets lined with decorative napkins:

Crispy Chicken Drummettes (page 289, served cold)

Individual containers of coleslaw

Roll

Fresh bunch of raw green beans wrapped in a ribbon

Small bag of chips

Old-Fashioned Jelly Roll (below)

Old-Fashioned Jelly Roll

5 eggs, separated

1 cup sugar

1 tablespoon lemon juice

2 tablespoons lemon zest

1 cup flour

1 cup raspberry (or other flavor) preserves

Confectioners' sugar

In a large bowl, beat egg yolks until frothy. Add sugar and beat.
Add juice and zest. Blend well. In a small bowl, beat egg whites

until stiff. Add flour and egg white alternately to batter, beating well after each addition. Pour into a jelly roll pan lined with waxed paper. Bake at 375° for 12 to 15 minutes. Turn out on a damp towel. Trim off the crusty edges and spread with jam. Roll up and cool. Sprinkle with confectioners' sugar and slice in 1- to 2-inch slices.

Yield: 12–16 servings

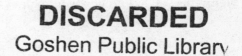

The ABC's of Getting Outside Help

This appendix makes getting additional help as easy as A, B, C. It is quite possible that even after reading this book, you have questions about your dairy-sensitive child's lifestyle or would like even more information and support. To help you, I have collected some resource information and divided it into three categories.

The letter A stands for associations and other health organizations that offer assistance for parents and children coping with milk-protein allergy, lactose intolerance, or other diseases that require the elimination of dairy foods from the diet. These organizations help by offering printed information, expert advice, support groups, or all three. Also included in this section are government and other regulatory agencies that deal with health-care issues regarding children. These may be of interest to parents who want to study current legislation and administrative regulations that affect their children in school or in other institutional settings.

Information found under the letter B includes books, newsletters, and other assorted pamphlets, which offer parenting advice and support. You will also find some specific information valuable for coping with allergic or food-intolerant children. Materials that relate to school issues are included in this section.

The letter C stands for the current products on the market that may serve your family well. This list includes several dairy-free food manufacturers, lactase enzyme product information, and names of other manufacturers that produce household items that will help relieve your child's allergic symptoms.

While these source lists are hardly exhaustive, I am hopeful that, with this information at hand, you will never again feel as though you are going through this all alone. Remember, there are millions of parents out there trying to raise healthy children without milk. They are succeeding with the support and advice of a variety of health organizations, national support groups, and a number of well-informed and sensitive physicians and dietitians—not to mention the essential help of food and other product manufacturers who are addressing the needs of dairy-sensitive children in so many ways. Your child's pediatrician, gastroenterologist, or allergist may have more names to add to these lists, or you can check your local library's reference section for additional help.

These lists include sources that I believe will be helpful to you and your child's individual challenges. You will see that I do not usually refer to any organization or book that is not grounded in careful scientific research and proven theories, although I do believe that alternative solutions to problems may be useful at times. In addition, these lists are in no way meant to be an endorsement of any product or a recommendation of any specific agency or individual. Please use this list merely as a guide to information sources and products that could be of value to you and your family. Additionally, information like this often goes quickly out of date, and if you find that some addresses or phone numbers are no longer available, I apologize for the inconvenience.

Furthermore, I always appreciate hearing from readers about their experiences (both good and bad) with organizations and professionals meant to serve the public. Please feel free to write to me and let me know how your problems were addressed. Send your letters to:

Jane Zukin c/o The Newsletter
PO Box 3129
Ann Arbor, MI 48106-3129

The A List: Associations and Organizations

Allergy and Asthma Network/Mothers of Asthmatics Inc.
3554 Chain Bridge Rd., Suite 200
Fairfax, VA 22030
703-385-4403
800-878-4403

Allergy Information Association
25 Poynter Dr., Room 7
Weston, Ontario M9R 1K8 Canada

American Academy of Allergy and Immunology
611 East Wells St.
Milwaukee, WI 53202
414-272-6071

American Allergy Association
PO Box 7273
Menlo Park, CA 94026
415-322-1663

American Celiac Society
58 Musano Ct.
West Orange, NJ 07052
201-325-8837

American Dietetic Association
430 North Michigan Ave.
Chicago, IL 60611

Association for the Care of Children's Health
7910 Woodmont Ave., Suite 300
Bethesda, MD 20814
301-654-6549

Asthma and Allergy Foundation
5410 Wilshire Blvd., Suite 1008
Los Angeles, CA 90036

Asthma and Allergy Foundation of America
1717 Massachusetts Ave. NW, Suite 305
Washington, DC 20036
202-265-0265

Canadian Coeliac/Sprue Association
PO Box 492
Kitchener, Ontario N2G 4A2 Canada

Celiac Sprue Association Inc./United States of America
PO Box 31700
Omaha, NE 68103-0700
402-558-0600

Center for Children with Chronic Illness and Disability
Box 721-UMHC
Harvard Street at East River Road
Minneapolis, MN 66566
612-626-4032

Center for Law and Education
955 Massachusetts Ave.
Cambridge, MA 02139

Child Care Law Center
22 Second St., Fifth Floor
San Francisco, CA 94105
415-495-5498

Crohn's and Colitis Foundation
444 Park Ave. South
New York, NY 10016-7374

Family Voices (This group advocates health-care reform.)
PO Box 769
Algodones, NM 87001

Federation for Children with Special Needs
95 Berkeley St.
Boston, MA 02166
617-482-2915

Food Allergy Network
4744 Holly Ave.
Fairfax, VA 22030-5647

Gluten Intolerance Group of North America
PO Box 23053
Seattle, WA 98102-0353
206-325-6980

Hood Center for Family Support (support for disabled teens)
Dartmouth-Hitchcock Medical Center
1 Medical Center Dr.
Lebanon, NH 03756

LaLeche League International
PO Box 1209
Franklin Park, IL 60131

Midwestern Celiac-Sprue Association
2313 Rocklyn Dr. #1
Des Moines, IA 50322

National Alliance for the Mentally Ill Children and Adolescents
      Network
2101 Wilson Blvd., Suite 30
Arlington, VA 22201
703-524-7600

National Institute of Allergy and Infectious Diseases
National Institutes of Health
Bethesda, MD 20205

National Association of School Nurses Inc.
Lamplighter Lane
PO Box 1300
Scarborough, ME 04074

National Center for Family-Centered Care
7910 Woodmont Ave., Suite 300
Bethesda, MD 20814
301-654-6549

National Center for Youth with Disabilities
Box 721-UMHC
Harvard Street at East River Road
Minneapolis, MN 55455
612-626-2825
800-333-6293

National Committee for Citizens in Education (advocate for
    parents rights in education)
800 Second St., Suite 8
Washington, DC 20002
202-408-0477
800-NETWORK

National Digestive Diseases Information Clearinghouse
2 Information Way
Bethesda, MD 20892-3570
301-654-3810

National Health Information Clearinghouse
PO Box 1133
Washington, DC 20013
800-336-4797

National Information Center for Children and Youth with
        Handicaps
PO Box 1492
Washington, DC 20013
800-999-5599

National Food Service Management Institute
University of Mississippi
PO Drawer 188
University, MS 38677-02188
601-232-7658

Nonprescription Drug Manufacturers Association
Office of Public Affairs
1150 Connecticut Ave. NW
Washington, DC 20036

Office on the Americans with Disabilities Act
Civil Rights Division
U.S. Department of Justice
PO Box 66118
Washington, DC 20035-6118
202-514-0301

Parent Information Center
Peer and Family Training Network Project on the ADA
PO Box 1422
Concord, NH 03302-1422
603-224-0402

Parent to Parent of Vermont (peer support)
1 Main Street
#69 Champlain Mill
Winooski, VT 05404
802-655-5290

Practical Allergy Research Foundation
PO Box 60
Buffalo, NY 14223-0060

Public Citizen Health Research Group
PO Box 19404
Washington, DC 20036

U.S. Department of Agriculture
Food and Nutrition Service
Room 304
10301 Baltimore Blvd.
Beltsville, MD 20705-2351

U.S. Department of Education
Office of Civil Rights
Washington, DC 20202-1328

U.S. Food and Drug Administration
5600 Fishers Lane
Bethesda, MD 20857

U.S.D.A. National Agricultural Library
NAL Building, Sixth Floor
10301 Baltimore Blvd.
Beltsville, MD 20705-2351
301-504-5994

U.S. Department of Health and Human Services
Public Health Service
Health Resources and Services Administration
Maternal and Child Health Bureau
Washington, DC 20857

The B List: Books, Newsletters, and Other Printed Matter

A-Z Guide to Your Child's Behavior
Faculty of the Children's National Medical Center
Perigee Books/Putnam Publishing Group, 1993

Allergy Control Products Catalog
28 High Ridge Rd.
Ridgefield, CT 06877

Allergy Hotline (Newsletter)
PO Box 161132
Altamonte Springs, FL 32716-1132
407-628-1377

Allergy Product Directory
PO Box 640
Menlo Park, CA 94026-0640
415-322-1663

Allergy Resource Products Limited Catalog
14319 63rd Ave.
Edmonton, Alberta T6H 1S3 Canada

Baby Eats!
Lois Smith
Berkley Books, 1994

Dairy-Free Cookbook
Jane Zukin
Prima Publishing, 1989

Dr. Spock's Baby and Child Care
Benjamin Spock, M.D., and Michael B. Rothenberg, M.D.
Pocket Books/Simon & Schuster Inc., 1992

Complete Book of Vitamins & Minerals
The Editors of *Consumer Guide*
Publications International, Ltd., 1993

Educational Rights of Children with Disabilities:
    A Primer for Advocates
Eileen L. Ordover and Kathleen B. Boundy
The Center for Law Education
955 Massachusetts Ave.
Cambridge, MA 02139
617-876-6611

Feed Me, I'm Yours
Vicki Lansky
Simon and Schuster, 1994

FDA Consumer
The Magazine of the U.S. FDA
5600 Fishers Lane
Rockville, MD 20857

Foods for Healthy Kids
Lendon Smith, M.D.
Berkley Books/McGraw-Hill Inc., 1984

Guidelines for Serving Students with Special Health Care Needs
Utah State Office of Education
Services for At-Risk Students Section
250 East 500 South
Salt Lake City, UT 84111
801-538-7778

Healthy Kids: The Key to Basics (information/consulting
    service)
Consultant: Ellie Goldberg, M.Ed.
79 Elmore St.
Newton, MA 02159-1137
617-965-9637

Improving Your Child's Behavior Chemistry
Lendon Smith, M.D.
Berkley Books/McGraw-Hill Inc.

Is This Your Child?
Doris J. Rapp, M.D., FAAA, FAAP
William Morrow, 1991

Lactose Intolerance Revised Edition
Merri Lou Dobler, M.S., R.D.
The American Dietetic Association
216 West Jackson Blvd.
Chicago, IL 60606-6995
312-899-0040

Milk-Free Holiday Cooking
Jane Zukin
Commercial Writing and Design, 1988

Newsletter for People with Lactose Intolerance and Milk Allergy
Published Bimonthly by Jane Zukin
PO Box 3129
Ann Arbor, MI 48106-3129
313-572-9134

Parents' Nutrition Book
Margaret McWilliams
John Wiley & Sons Inc., 1986

Planning for Life after High School: A Handbook of
    Information and Resources for Families and Young Adults
    with Disabilities
Full Citizenship Inc.
211 East Eighth, Suite F
Lawrence, KS 66044
913-749-0603

School Nurses Source Book of Individualized Healthcare Plans
MaryKay B. Haas, et al
Sunrise River Press
11481 Kost Dam Rd.
North Branch, MN 55056
800-551-4754

Serving Students with Special Health Care Needs
Connecticut Department of Education
State Office Building, Room 304
PO Box 2219
Hartford, CT 06145-2219
203-566-5677

The Impossible Child
Doris J. Rapp, M.D., FAAA, FAAP
Practical Allergy Research Foundation, 1986

The Taming of the C.A.N.D.Y. Monster
A Cookbook to Get Kids to Eat Less Junk Food
Vicki Lansky
The Book Peddlers, 1988

Touchpoints: The Essential Reference
T. Berry Brazelton, M.D.
Addison-Wesley Publishing Company, 1992

Your Baby & Child From Birth to Age Five
Penelope Leach, Ph.D.
Alfred A. Knopf, 1994

The C List: Current Products on the Market

Dairy-Free and Other Specialty Food Products

Allergy Resources
PO Box 888
264 Brookridge
Palmer Lake, CA 80133
800-USE-FLAX

Allergy Resources
62 Firwood Rd.
Port Washington, NY 11050
516-767-2000

Amaranth Flour
Illinois Amaranth Company
PO Box 464
Mundelein, IL 60060
312-566-4794

Amaranth Flour
Post Rock Natural Grains
RT 1 Box 24
Luray, KS 67649

Arrowhead Mills Inc.
PO Box 866
Hereford, TX 79045
806-364-0730

Azymaya Inc. (tofu products)
1575 Burke Ave.
San Francisco, CA 94124

Bio-Tech Systems
PO Box 25380
Chicago, IL 60625
800-621-5545

Brightsong Light Foods (nondairy frozen desserts)
PO Box 2536
Petaluma, CA 94953

Bronson Pharmaceuticals
4526 Rinetti Lane
La Cañada, CA 91011
800-521-3323

Butte Creek Mill
PO Box 561
Eagle Point, OR 97524
503-826-3531

Chicago Dietetic Supply
405 E. Shawmut Ave.
PO Box 40
La Grange, IL 60525
312-352-6900

Chico-San Inc.
PO Box 810
Chico, CA 95927
916-891-6271

Clear Eyes Natural Foods
RD 1 Box 89
Savannah, NY 13146-9790
315-365-2816

Colombo Breezer (nondairy soft serve)
General Mills Corporation
PO Box 1113
Minneapolis, MN 55440
612-540-7784

Dean Foods Lactose-Reduced Milk
3600 River Rd.
Franklin Park, IL 60131

Deer Valley Farm
RD 1
Guillford, NY 13780
607-764-8556

Dietary Specialties Inc.
PO Box 227
Rochester, NY 14601

Dole Fruit Sorbet
Castle and Cook Inc.
50 California St.
San Francisco, CA 94111

Ecology Box (organic baby food)
425 East Washington #202
Ann Arbor, MI 48104
313-662-9131

Edensoy (soy products)
Eden Foods
701 Tecumseh Rd.
Clinton, MI 49236

Elam's
2625 Gardner Rd.
Broadview, IL 60153
708-865-1612

Ener-G Foods Inc.
PO Box 24723
Seattle, WA 98124

GFA Brands
Smart Beat Products
PO Box 397
Cresskill, NJ 07626-0397
201-568-9300

General Foods Consumer Center
250 North St.
White Plains, NY 10625
800-431-1001

General Mills Inc.
9200 Wayzata Blvd.
Minneapolis, MN 55440

General Nutrition Corporation
921 Penn Ave.
Pittsburgh, PA 15222

Glenn Foods
112 Hudson St.
Copiague, NY 11728

Good Food Guide
Natural Organic Farmers Association
RD 1 Box 134 A
Port Crane, NY 13833
607-648-5557

Hain's Safflower Margarine
Hain's Pure Food Company
PO Box 54841 Terminal Annex
13660 South Figueroa St.
Los Angeles, CA 90061

Health Valley Foods Inc. (Soy-Moo milk)
700 Union St.
Montebello, CA 90604

Heinz U.S.A.
Consumer Relations Department
Pittsburgh, PA 15230

Ice Bean Frozen Dessert
Farm Foods Inc.
123 South St.
Oyster Bay, NY 11771

Kingsmill Foods Company Ltd. (lactase enzyme/lactose-
    reduced milk)
1399 Kennedy Rd., Unit 17
Scarborough, Ontario M1P 2L6 Canada

Lifestream Natural Foods Ltd.
12411 Vulcan Way
Richmont, British Columbia V6V 1J7 Canada

Loma Linda Foods (soy products)
11503 Pierce St.
Riverside, CA 92515

Lotus Bakery (specialty baked goods)
2201 S. Bluebell Dr.
Santa Rosa, CA 95401

Mama Tish's Gourmet Sorbetto (sorbet)
5245 N. Rose St.
Rosemont, IL 60018

Manischewitz Food Products (kosher/parve foods)
1 Manischewitz Plaza
Jersey City, NJ 07302

Mar-Parv Margarine
The Miami Margarine Company
Cincinnati, OH 45217

Med-Diet Laboratories Inc. (specialty foods)
1415 Fairfield Rd. S
PO Box 27251
Golden Valley, MN 55427

Mocha Mix Non-Dairy Creamer
Presto Food Products
PO Box 584
Industry, CA 91747-0584

Morinaga Nutritional Foods Inc. (tofu products)
5800 S. Eastern Ave. #270
Los Angeles, CA 90040

Natural and Kosher Foods Inc. (kosher/parve foods)
14110 S. Broadway
Los Angeles, CA 90061

Quaker Oats Company
Merchandise Mart Plaza
Chicago, IL 60654

Rice Dream
Imagine Foods Inc.
Jamestown, MO 65046

Rich Products Corporation (nondairy creamer/whipped cream)
1150 Niagara St.
Buffalo, NY 14240

Sharon's Finest
PO Box 5020
Santa Rosa, CA 95402-5020
707-544-4635

Shiloh Farms
PO Box 97
Sulfur Springs, AR 72768
501-298-3297

Special Foods
9207 Shotgun Ct.
Springfield, VA 22153
703-644-0991

Sun Savory Foods Inc.
RD 5 Box 5327
Newton, NJ 07860
201-579-4888

This Is Blis (nondairy soft serve)
Deirdre Murphy/Cone-Ucopia Inc.
8522 National Blvd.
Culver City, CA 90232-2454
800-892-5283

Tofulite Frozen Dessert
Barricini Foods Inc.
123 South St.
Oyster Bay, NY 11771

Tofu Pops
Tuscan Dairies
750 Union
Union, NY 07083

Tofutti/Tofutti Lite Frozen Dessert
Tofu Time Inc.
1638 63rd St.
Brooklyn, NY 11204

Vitamite Lactose-Free Non-Dairy Beverage
Diehl Specialities International
24 N. Clinton St.
Defiance, OH 43512-1899
800-443-3930

Vitasoy (soy products)
99 Park Lane
Brisbane, CA 94005
415-467-8888

Vita-Wheat Baked Products Inc. (specialty baked goods)
1839 Hamilton Rd.
Ferndale, MI 48220

Worthington Foods Inc. (soy products)
900 Proprietors Rd.
Worthington, OH 43085

Lactase-Enzyme Products

Dairy Ease
Winthrop Consumer Products
90 Park Ave.
New York, NY 10016
800-233-7500

Good Sense Lactase Enzyme
Bob Leonard
PO Box 6691 Dept. B
New York, NY 10128
212-831-6612

LactAid Inc. (lactase enzyme/lactose-reduced milk and cheese)
800-LACTAID

Lactose Solution Enzyme
Bioenergy Nutrients
6565 Odell Place
Boulder, CO 80301-3330

Lactozyme
Schiff Bio-Foods
121 Moonachie Ave.
Moonachie, NJ 07074

Lactrase Enzyme
Schwarz Pharma/Kremers Urban Company
PO Box 2038
Milwaukee, WI 53201
800-558-5114

Milk-Gest
Nulife Inc.
Orange, CA 92667

Natural Brand Milk Digestant Tablet
Natural Sales Company
PO Box 25
Pittsburgh, PA 15230

Super Milk Digestant
Malabar Formulas
28537 Nuevo Valley Dr.
PO Box 3
Nuevo, CA 92367

Allergy Relief Products

AllerGard
1645 SW 41st St.
Topeka, KA 66609
913-267-9333

Allergy Clean Environments
125 Haddon Ave.
Haddon Heights, NJ 08035
800-882-4110

Allergy Control Products
96 Danbury Rd.
Ridgefield, CT 06887
800-442-3878

Allergy Relief Products
246-08 Jericho Turnpike
Floral Park, NY 11001
800-862-5155

Bio-Tech Systems
PO Box 25380
Chicago, IL 60625

"Feed Me Dairy Free" Products
T-Shirts/Recipe Cards/Dairy-Free Labeling Stickers
c/o The Newsletter
PO Box 3129
Ann Arbor, MI 48106-3129
313-572-9134

Infolert Badges (badges worn by children with food allergies)
27068 La Paz #324
Laguna Hills, CA 92656
714-454-8809

Living Source (allergy products directory)
3500 MacArthur Dr.
Waco, TX 76708
817-756-6341

National Allergy Supply
4579 Georgia Hwy 120
PO Box 1658
Duluth, GA 30136
800-522-1448

Pathway (custom hypoallergenic pharmaceuticals)
5414 W. Cedar Ln.
Bethesda, MD 20814
301-530-1112
800-889-9160

Professional Compounding Centers of America (PCCA)
(custom hypoallergenic pharmaceuticals)
800-331-2498

Sierra Group for Environmental Products Inc.
433 Rivers Edge Ct.
Nishawake, IN 46544
800-234-9517

Bibliography

The following list of references represents approximately half of the sources used in the development of this book; these have been selected for notation here based on their specific relevance to the subject of dairy sensitivity in infants and children.

Books

Appleton, Nancy. *Healthy Bones.* Garden City Park: Avery Publishing Group, 1991.

Brazelton, T. Berry, M.D. *Touchpoints.* New York: Addison-Wesley Publishing Company, 1992.

Delmont, J., ed. *Milk Intolerances and Rejection.* London: Karger, 1983.

Dodson, Fitzhugh. *How To Parent.* New York: Penguin Group, Signet, 1971.

Favaro, Peter. *Smart Parenting.* Chicago: Contemporary Books, 1994.

Galambos, John T., M.D. and Theodore Hersh, M.D. *Digestive Diseases.* Boston: Butterworths, 1983.

Gasbarro, Ron. *Prescription Drugs.* Springhouse: American Health Family Institute/Springhouse Corporation, 1986.

Hsia, David Yi-Yung, M.D. *Galactosemia.* Springfield: Charles C. Thomas Publisher, 1969.

Janowitz, Henry D., M.D. *Your Gut Feelings.* New York: Oxford University Press, 1987.

Lawrence, Ruth A., M.D. *Breastfeeding: A Guide for the Medical Profession.* Rochester, NY: C. V. Mosby Company, 1989.

Leach, Penelope. *Your Baby & Child.* New York: Alfred A. Knopf, 1994.

Long, James W., M.D., and James J. Rybacki. *The Essential Guide to Prescription Drugs 1994.* New York: HarperCollins Publishers, Inc, 1994.

McWilliams, Margaret. *The Parents' Nutrition Book.* New York: John Wiley & Sons, Inc, 1986.

Mrazek, David, M.D., and William Garrison. *A–Z Guide to Your Child's Behavior.* New York: Putnam Publishing Group, Perigee Books, 1993.

Natow, Annette, and Jo-Ann Heslin. *No-Nonsense Nutrition for Kids.* New York: Simon & Schuster, Inc., Pocket Books, 1985.

Netzer, Corinne T. *The Complete Book of Food Counts.* New York: Dell Publishing, 1991.

Paige, David M., M.D., and Theodore M. Bayless, M.D. *Lactose Digestion: Clinical and Nutritional Implications.* Baltimore: Johns Hopkins University Press, 1981.

Rapp, Doris, M.D. *Is This Your Child?* New York: William Morrow, Quill, 1991.

——. *The Impossible Child.* Buffalo: Practical Allergy Research Foundation, 1986.

Robinson, Corinne H. *Normal and Therapeutic Nutrition*, 14th ed. New York: Macmillan Publishing Co., Inc, 1972.

Smith, Lendon, M.D. *Foods for Healthy Kids.* New York: Berkley Books, published by arrangement with McGraw-Hill Inc, 1981.

——. *Improving Your Child's Behavior Chemistry.* New York: Berkley Books, published by arrangement with McGraw-Hill Inc.

Smith, Lois. *Baby Eats!* New York: Berkley Books, 1994.

Spock, Benjamin, M.D., and Michael B. Rothenberg, M.D. *Dr. Spock's Baby and Child Care.* New York: Simon & Schuster, Inc., Pocket Books, 1992.

Walker, W. Allan, M.D., and John B. Watkins, M.D. *Nutrition in Pediatrics.* Boston: Little Brown & Co., 1985.

Whitehead, William, M.D. and Marvin M. Schuster, M.D. *Gastrointestinal Disorders: Behavioral and Psychological Basis for Treatment.* New York: Harcourt Brace Jovanovich Publishers, Academic Press Inc., 1985.

Whitlock, Evelyn P., M.D. *The Calcium Plus Workbook.* New Canaan, CT: Keats Publishing, Inc., 1988.

Articles

Bayless, Theodore, M.D. "Recognition of Lactose Intolerance." *Hospital Practice* (October 1976): 97–101.

Bayless, Theodore, M.D., Irwin H. Rosenberg, M.D., and W. Allan Walker, M.D. "When To Suspect Lactose Intolerance." *Patient Care* (September 30, 1987): 136–47.

Debrovner, Diane. "Does Milk Shake You Up?" *American Druggist* (September 1993): 42–49.

Goldberg, Ellie. "Students with Food Allergies: What Do the Laws Say." *Food Allergy News* (August–September 1992).

Hingley, Audrey T. "Food Allergies: When Eating Is Risky." *FDA Consumer* (December 1993): 27–31.

Hunter, Beatrice Trum. "Lactose Intolerance." *Consumers' Research* (March 1986): 8–9.

Kleiner, Susan. "Sidestepping Food Sensitivities." *The Physician and Sports Medicine* (March 1993): 59–60.

Kurtzweil, Paula. "Food Label Close-Up." *FDA Consumer* (April 1994): 15–19.

Montes, Ramon, M.D., and Jay Perman, M.D., "Lactose Intolerance: Pinpointing the Source of Nonspecific Gastrointestinal Symptoms." *Postgraduate Medicine* (June 1991): 175–84.

Pearce, Janet. "Milk: No Longer a Sacred Cow." *Family Health* (April 4, 1973): 28.

Prescott, Bonnie. "Milk's Great White Way." *Health* (September 1987): 71–73.

Quint, Laurie. "The New Calcium Crop." *Eater's Digest* (October 1986): 10–11.

Stehlin, Dori. "Feeding Baby: Nature and Nurture." *FDA Consumer* (September 1993).

Studies

Abramowitz, A., et al. "Two-Hour Lactose Breath Hydrogen Test." *Journal of Pediatric Gastroenterology & Nutrition* (January 1986): 130–33.

Arola, H., et al. "Strip Test Is Reliable in Common Prevalences of Hypolactasia." *Scandanavian Journal of Gastroenterology* (May 1987): 509–12.

Bahna, S. L. "New Aspects of Diagnosis of Milk Allergy in Children." *Allergy Proceedings* (July–August 1991): 217–20.

Biller, Jeffrey, et al. "Efficacy of Lactase-Treated Milk for Lactose-Intolerant Pediatric Patients." *The Journal of Pediatrics* (July 1987): 91–94.

Bottaro, G., et al. "Comparison of Two Methods to Determine Beta-Lactoglobulin Antibodies in Children with Cow's Milk Protein Intolerance." *Pediatria Medica a Chirurgica* (January–February 1992): 27–30.

Bottaro, G., et al. "Significance of Milk Antibodies in Cow's Milk Protein Intolerance." *Pediatria Medica a Chirurgica* (January–February 1992): 21–25.

Brand, J. C., et al. "Lactase Deficiency in Australian School Children." *Medical Journal of Australia* (October 6, 1986): 318–22.

Bujanover, Y., et al. "Lactose Malabsorption in Israeli Children." *Israel Journal of Medical Sciences* (January 1985): 32–35.

Campbell, J. P. "Dietary Treatment of Infant Colic: A Double-Blind Study." *Journal of the Royal College of General Practitioners* (January 1989).

Casimir, G. J., et al. "Maternal Immune Status Against Beta-Lactoglobulin and Cow Milk Allergy in the Infant." *Annals of Allergy* (December 1989): 517–19.

Ceriani, R., et al. "Lactose Malabsorption and Recurrent Abdominal Pain in Italian Children." *Journal of Pediatric Gastroenterology & Nutrition* (November–December 1988): 852–57.

Enck, P., et al. "Lactase Deficiency and Lactose Malabsorption: A Review." *Zeitschrift für Gastroenterologie* (March 1986): 125–34.

Hill, D. J., et al. "Clinical Manifestations of Cow's Milk Allergy in Childhood. II The Diagnostic Value of Skin Tests and RAST." *Clinical Allergy* (September 1988): 481–90.

Hill, D. J., et al. "Recovery from Milk Allergy in Early Childhood: Antibody Studies." *Journal of Pediatrics* (May 1989): 761–66.

Hill, S. M., et al. "Cow's Milk Sensitive Enteropathy in Cystic Fibrosis." *Archives of Disease in Childhood* (September 1989): 1251–55.

Host, A., et al. "A Prospective Study of Cow's Milk Allergy in Exclusively Breast-Fed Infants." *Acta Paediatrica Scandinavica* (September 1988): 663–70.

Host, A., et al. "Allergic Reactions to Raw, Pasteurized, and Homogenized/Pasteurized Cow Milk: A Comparison." *Allergy* (February 1988): 113–18.

Husby, S., et al. "Infants and Children with Cow Milk Allergy/Intolerance. Investigation of the Uptake of Cow Milk Protein and Activation of the Complement System." *Allergy* (October 1990): Pages 547–51.

Iacono, S., et al. "Severe Infantile Colic and Food Intolerance: A Long-Term Prospective Study." *Journal of Pediatric Gastroenterology & Nutrition* (April 1991): 332–35.

Iyngkaran, N., et al. "Causative Effect of Cow's Milk Protein and Soy Protein on Progressive Small Bowel Mucosal Damage." *Journal of Gastroenterology & Hepatology* (March–April 1989): 127–36.

Johnson, Ronald C., et al. "Ethnic, Familial and Environmental Influences on Lactose Intolerance." *Human Biology* (May 1984): 307–16.

Kahn, Al, et al. "Milk Intolerance in Children with Persistent Sleeplessness: A Prospective Double-Blind Crossover Evaluation." *Pediatrics* (October 1989): 595–603.

Lifschitz, C. H., et al. "Absorption and Tolerance of Lactose in Infants Recovering from Severe Diarrhea." *Journal of Pediatric Gastroenterology & Nutrition* (December 1985): 942–48.

Lifschitz, C. H., et al. "Infant Absorption and Tolerance of Lactose." *Journal of Pediatric Gastroenterologic Nutrition* (November 6, 1985): 944–48.

Lloyd, T., et al. *Journal of American Medical Association* (August 1993): 270.

Martini, M. C., et al. "Lactose Digestion from Frozen Yogurts, Ice Milk, and Ice Cream by Lactase-Deficient Persons." *American Journal of Clinical Nutrition* (October 1987): 636–40.

Martini, M. C., et al. "Reduced Intolerance Symptoms from Lactose Consumed During a Meal." *American Journal of Clinical Nutrition* (January 1988): 57–60.

McDonough, F. E., et al. "Modification of Sweet Acidophilus Milk to Improve Utilization by Lactose-Intolerant Persons." *American Journal of Clinical Nutrition* (March 1987): 570–74.

Mojsoski, N. "Bronchial Asthma and Methomoglobinemia Caused by Milk Allergy." *Plucne Bolesti* (January–June 1991): 83–85.

Moore, D. J., et al. "Breath Hydrogen Response to Milk Containing Lactose in Colicky and Noncolicky Infants." *Journal of Pediatrics* (August 1989): 333–34.

Moskovitz, M., et al. "Does Oral Enzyme Replacement Therapy Reverse Intestinal Lactose Malabsorption?" *American Journal of Gastroenterology* (July 1987): 632–35.

Salazar, de Sousa J., et al. "Cow's Milk Protein-Sensitive Enteropathy: Number and Timing of Biopsies for Diagnosis." *Journal of Pediatric Gastroenterology & Nutrition"* (March–April 1986).

Samson, H. A., et al. "Safety of Casein Hydrolysate Formula in Children with Cow Milk Allergy." *Journal of Pediatrics* (April 1991): 520–25.

Savilahti, E., et al. "Low Colostral IgA Associated with Cow's Milk Allergy." *Acta Paediatrica Scandinavica* (December 1991): 1207–13.

Scrimsaw, N. S., et al. "Lactose Intolerance and Milk Consumption: Myths and Realities." *Archivos Latinoamericanos de Nutricion* (September 1988): 543–67.

Ting, C. W., et al. "Developmental Changes of Lactose Malabsorption in Normal Chinese Children: A Study Using Breath Hydrogen Test with a Physiological Dose of Lactose." *Journal of Pediatric Gastroenterology & Nutrition* (November–December 1988): 848–51.

Tolbloom, J. J., et al. "Incomplete Lactose Absorption from Breast Milk During Acute Gastroenteritis." *Acta Paediatrica Scandinavica* (January 1986): 151–55.

Welsh, Jack D., M.D. "Diet Therapy in Adult Lactose Malabsorption: Present Practices." *The American Journal of Clinical Nutrition* (April 1978): 592–96.

Pamphlets/Periodicals

Allergy Foundation of Canada. *A Guide to Living with Milk Allergy.* Saskatoon, 1978

American Allergy Association. *Allergy Products Directory.* Menlo Park, 1987.

American Dietetic Association. *Labeling Logic.* Chicago.

———. *Lactose Intolerance.* Chicago, 1991.

American Family Physician. *Cow's Milk Intolerance and Sleeplessness in Children.* July 1990.

———. *Lactose Malabsorption in Infants with Colic.* July 1989.

American Institute for Cancer Research Newsletter. *Good Nutrition Starts at Home.* Washington, D.C., Fall 1989.

American Institute for Cancer Research. *Infant Nutrition: Sound Eating Habits Start Early.* Washington, D.C.

Division of Health: Wisconsin Department of Health and Social Services. *Nutrition Newsletter for Consultant Dietitians.* July–August–September 1978.

Gerber Products Company. *Dietary Guidelines for Infants.* Fremont, Michigan, 1989.

Harvard Health Letter. *Unkind Milk.* Boston, October 1993.

Healthy Kids: The Key to Basics. *Educational Planning for Students with Chronic Health Conditions.* Newton, MA.

Mayo Clinic Health Letter. *Allergy Tests: Some Newer Methods Are More Hype Than Help.* Rochester, March 1989.

National Digestive Disease Information Clearinghouse. *Lactose Intolerance: Important Information for You and Your Family.* Washington, D.C., 1987.

Nutrition Reviews. *Efficacy of Exogenous Lactase for Lactose Intolerance.* April 1988.

Tufts University Diet & Nutrition Letter. *Colicky Babies and Breast Milk.* New York, November 1983.

———. *Getting around a Baby's Allergy to Cow's Milk.* New York, August 1987.

———. *Most Children Outgrow Early Food Allergies.* New York, September 1988.

———. *The Best Way to Treat Your Child's Diarrhea.* New York, April 1990.

University of California Berkeley Wellness Letter. *Diagnosing Food Allergies.* Berkeley, May 1992.

———. *Maximizing Your Minerals.* Berkeley, August 1992.

———. *The Lactase Craze.* Berkeley, November 1993.

U.S. Department of Health and Human Services. *Child Health USA '92.* Washington, D.C., March 1993.

———. *Child Health Guide.* Washington, D.C., June 1994.

———. *The Surgeon General's Report on Nutrition and Health.* Washington, D.C., 1988.

World Health Organization. *Lactose Malabsorption in Relation to Health Promotion.* June 1985.

Index